Housing Risks and Homelessness Among the Urban Elderly

Housing Risks and Homelessness Among the Urban Elderly

Sharon M. Keigher
Editor

The Haworth Press
New York • London • Sydney

Housing Risks and Homelessness Among the Urban Elderly has also been published as the *Journal of Housing for the Elderly,* Volume 8, Number 1 1991.

The Haworth Press, Inc. 10 Alice Street, Binghamton, NY 13904-1580
EUROSPAN/Haworth, 3 Henrietta Street, London WC2E 8LU England
ASTAM/Haworth, 162-168 Parramatta Road, Stanmore, N.S.W. 2048 Australia

Library of Congress Cataloging-in-Publication Data

Housing risks and homelessness among the urban elderly / Sharon M. Keigher, editor.
p. cm.
"Has also been published as Journal of housing for the elderly, volume 8, number 1, 1991 – T.p. verso.
ISBN 1-56024-165-9 (acid free paper)
1. Aged – Housing – United States. 2. Homeless persons – Housing – United States. 3. Urban poor – Housing – United States. 4. Aged – Illinois – Chicago – Social conditions – Case studies. 5. Aged – Housing – Illinois – Chicago – Case studies. I. Keigher, Sharon Marie, 1947–
HV1461.H69 1991
363.5'946'0973 – dc20 91-22606
CIP

Housing Risks and Homelessness Among the Urban Elderly

CONTENTS

PART II: THE HOMELESS AND NEAR-HOMELESS ELDERLY AND HOW THEY COPE

PART IV: THE HUMAN COST

ABOUT THE EDITOR

Sharon Keigher, PhD, ACSW, is Associate Professor of Social Work at the University of Michigan, Ann Arbor. A social worker for twenty years, she has worked in corrections, mental health, and community development and in state government as a budget analyst and social service planner. Dr. Keigher is currently a consultant to the Older Women's League, studying the implications of the growing crisis in affordability of housing for the elderly as it affects aging women. She is also studying compensation schemes for family and informal care of the elderly. Dr. Keigher has published her research in a variety of journals and has given presentations for the Gerotological Society of America and the American Society on Aging. She received her doctorate in social welfare policy from the University of Chicago School of Social Service Administration in 1985.

ALL HAWORTH BOOKS & JOURNALS
ARE PRINTED ON CERTIFIED
ACID-FREE PAPER

Preface

The Growth and Significance of Housing Problems Among Older Urban Americans

Housing problems and homelessness among the elderly are problems which will require substantial attention in the 1990s. High rents, deteriorating housing conditions, and an increasing shortage of housing options are problems which affect a significant proportion of elders. The growing rate of homelessness among the elderly, although small relative to other groups in the population, is likely to be of continual concern.

Homelessness is a broad term encompassing persons with a variety of needs and circumstances. As each city "discovers" homelessness on its own, the term's definition takes on a variety of local manifestations. Discourse is constrained by the very social construction of the term "homelessness" which suggests a condition persons have or do not have (Berman, Iris, Keigher, in press), rather than a range or continuum of conditions of risk. Studies in America are constrained by traditional views of the underclass, as well as by the wide variance in local history, economic development, and demographics. The wide range of risky circumstances and housing problems which can capture elderly persons are difficult to analyze comprehensively. Many forces are relatively new and poorly documented.

Concomitant with and related to homelessness, the 1980s saw a resurgence in poverty among certain vulnerable and dependent groups, including some of the aged. As in any time when the middle class begins to slip in status, society has tended to respond to the extreme and most visible victims, often ignoring the full range of difficulties felt by all who are dislocated.

The "traditional homeless," typically older single and alcoholic men living in the Boweries and Skid Rows of our cities, have been studied for years. But "new" classes of the "deserving" poor are emerging. The "new homeless" include the elderly, "shopping bag ladies," drug abusers, persons with AIDS, and the mentally disabled, as well as young unemployed minority males, women and children. The need is great to understand the circumstances that threaten these individuals in order to prevent them. Yet, little is known about who such persons are, how they become homeless, or their prospects for longevity, much less how they subsist, their marginal opportunities and their prospects of finding replacement housing. The very poor elderly would seem to be especially at risk, given that as a cohort they experience fixed incomes, health problems, and losses of social support with advancing age. But it is not so easy to discern how homelessness "happens."

This special volume casts a wide net around the housing problems that are related to homelessness and near homelessness among the very low-income urban elderly. The majority of this volume reports on a comprehensive study of housing related problems of the elderly conducted by Sharon Keigher, Rebecca Berman and Sadelle Greenblatt in Chicago in 1988. The Housing Risks of the Elderly Project examined the problems of a broad cross section of elders seen briefly by a city emergency service agency. These chapters blend both quantitative and qualitative analyses of data gathered on 156 older Chicagoans. The goal is to understand how housing related problems and substandard residences lead to homelessness as well as preventable death and institutionalization.

Part I establishes the context and significance of housing problems for the elderly in the current political environment. Chapter 1 documents the extreme erosion of publically supported housing options for the elderly that has occurred in the 1980s, a spiraling vortex of budget cutbacks, scandals and decline of public confidence capped off with the particularly symbolic McKinney Homelessness Assistance Act. This erosion is matched in economically healthy cities by concomitant erosion of affordable private market housing stock. In this context in 1987 the present study commenced. Chapter 2 outlines the research goals, objectives and methodological approach of the Chicago study.

Part II of this volume uses a random sample of Chicago elders who have experienced emergencies to identify characteristics of the homeless and near homeless and how they appear to be coping with their situations. In this section the Chicago data is supplemented with data from Detroit. In Chapter 3 Keigher and Greenblatt describe the Emergency Service clients, their problems, and the services they utilize as documented in city emergency agency records. The authors then describe the levels of need and impairment of the interviewed clients. They compare those reported to be in need of temporary housing with those who were reported to be living in deplorable housing conditions and those living in SROs. They further compare those who have experienced homelessness with those who were never homeless, critically assessing where clients "ended up" since their emergency. Three factors are identified that appear to be especially salient to the vulnerability of the elderly and significantly correlated with having ever been homeless, with a summary of relevant findings and conclusions appearing at the end of this chapter. Chapter 3 thus characterizes statistically the kind of housing problem trajectories of elderly person who have experienced crises which are described qualitatively and graphically in later chapters.

The Chicago study's method is counterbalanced and supplemented by Richard Douglass and Ben Hodgkins' report of a field survey of the elderly homeless of Detroit, where many of the demographics of the elderly are similar. In contrast to the Chicago study's method, this study used the standard "street survey" sampling design to reach the traditional homeless. (Because individuals with a history of long term homelessness are largely invisible to traditional service agencies, such individuals were those least likely to be identified and located in the Chicago study.) Douglass and Hodgkins highlight the unique backgrounds of long term homeless elders related to their racial and socioeconomic characteristics. They have some characteristics that appear to be very different from the short term homeless and those who avoid homelessness. In some ways, however, they are indistinguishable from the elders with other housing problems found in the Chicago data, especially those living in single room occupancy hotels (SRO's). Racial differences with this homeless sample are suggestive of important environmental factors that merit further study.

In Chapter 5 Keigher and Berman present a qualitative analysis of some typical ES housing risk clients by describing their housing histories retrospectively. Client types include the brief and never homeless, the long term "chronically undomiciled" and those pathologically attached to unsafe or unassisted places. The vignettes focus on clients' coping capacities and the patterns of their residential moves, preliminarily assessing the organization of their lives and their attachments. The analysis identifies some key precipitants that lead to loss of elders' homes and the unique ways they cope with dislocation.

Part III of this volume highlights the special place of certain types of housing that serves very low income elders, with particular emphasis on SRO hotels. In Chapter 6, Beverly Ovrebo, Meredith Minkler and Petra Liljestrand discuss the importance of SRO housing for poor and marginally functioning elders. The authors chronicle the precipitous decline in the national supply of this resource, and note the effects of this erosion on the housing options for poor elders. Preservation of SROs is critical, especially to elderly residents who have resided in them for a very long time, but also for the marginally functioning and constantly transient elderly (such as those discussed by Douglass & Hodginson in Chapter 4). Both groups find accessible, convenient, private and affordable refuge there.

Chapters 7 and 8 report on the observed effects of the erosion of this cheap housing for poor elders in Chicago. Chapter 7 presents findings of a survey of 27 SROs and discusses the implications of the demise of this shrinking resource for elders in selected parts of the city. Chapter 8 discusses the unique strengths of this autonomous yet supportive environment for some older persons and the lessons that residents offer for effective service delivery. Suggestions for preservation and enhancement of such settings is also discussed.

Comparison of the emergency service user sample with the sample of SRO residents reveals areas of severe vulnerability and risk among the emergency service users which are at least partially compensated for in congregate housing settings such as SROs. Generalizable findings and conclusions that might predict for homelessness or becoming institutionalized, however, are modest and only account for a small proportion of the variation found that distinguish the ever homeless from the never homeless.

The last article in this volume, Chapter 9, addresses the risk factors identified among the elderly that can lead to loss of a home and the implications of these findings for more appropriate social services, as well as the growing desperation of elders and service providers facing a shrinking supply of low income housing options. This chapter concludes that low-income elderly persons who have suffered housing losses and housing related problems have very special needs for intensive help and effective interventions, problems which would be more effectively served through prevention programs. Outreach and assistance would be more acceptable to seniors if it were more available, adaptive and supported by a partnership of both agencies and casual helpers in neighborhoods. Appendix A presents the methodology and design of the data gathering and analysis.

Together these articles paint a disturbing picture of situations that should not have arisen at all if our nation's "safety net" were really working. Our nation could, and we believe must, do better in its commitment to these elderly people in the future. With the benefit of their observations and insights in these findings, we can see how housing and housing assistance could be provided in more humane and decent ways. Our nation's dismal housing policy record of the 1980s needs to be replaced soon with a commitment to housing everyone, thus *including* people "at risk" rather than targeting only those who are "worst off." If it is not, the preventable sadness and squalor, costly trauma and illness, and needless dislocation presented here will only grow worse throughout the 1990s.

Sharon M. Keigher, PhD

Acknowledgements

The majority of this volume reports on research by the Housing Risks of the Elderly Project conducted in Chicago in 1988. This project was supported by grants from the Retirement Research Foundation and the Robert Wood Johnson Foundation, and was conducted under auspices of the University of Michigan School of Social Work and sponsorship of the Metropolitan Chicago Coalition on Aging. A pilot study which initiated this study was conducted in 1987 with support of a Gerontological Society of America Postdoctoral Fellowship to the principal investigator and sponsorship by the Chicago Department of Aging and Disability. While the authors are immensely grateful to all the above sponsors and funders, our findings and conclusions should in no way be taken to reflect the positions or agreement of any of them as individuals or as agencies.

Several people who are not mentioned in the individual chapters to follow gave valuable and irreplaceable support to the Housing Risks of the Elderly Project in many ways. Special appreciation is due to Rosemary Gemperle and Renee Lumpkin of the Chicago Department of Aging and Disability whose vision and commitment started this project; to Ron Elling and all the staff at the Metropolitan Chicago Coalition on Aging whose flexibility and advice facilitated its implementation; and to all the staff at the Chicago Department of Human Services who were extraordinarily cooperative, given their own pressures.

More than anything else we are grateful to the older persons described in these chapters who talked with us. They have generously shared their lives, their feelings and their experiences – their pain, frustration, and sometimes desperation – because they believed that telling us would shed light on the housing problems of older Americans and *might* help resolve them for *other* people . . . someday. They asked little or nothing for themselves and often, only asked to be left alone. We believe, however, that a humane society would assure them more decent basic provisions than this.

PART I: A NATIONAL CRISIS

Chapter 1

Growing Housing Hardship Among the Elderly

Sharon M. Keigher
with Faith Pratt

SUMMARY. This chapter overviews the current housing context facing the elderly in terms of the increasing pressures on economically and vulnerable elders. The focus is on forces that aggravate the vulnerabilities especially of the very poor and very old who live alone in large urban environments. Key trends that have been of growing significance during the 1980s are reviewed with focus on the erosion of federally subsidized housing programs for the aging. This is followed by a discussion of the forces affecting the availability of affordable housing and the precipitants of homelessness among elders in one major city, Chicago.

The 1980s saw a startling erosion of America's commitment to the provision of housing for low income people as a national goal. As the number of elders gradually grows and projections of growth continue well into the 21st century, the nation's infrastructure of basic housing resources has begun to substantially erode. It is significant that homelessness has grown so dramatically in the 1980s and is expected to continue to grow into the foreseeable future (U.S. Conference of Mayors, 1986 & 1987; National Coalition of the Homeless; Congressional Budget Office, 1988). Homelessness appears to be increasing at least as fast among the elderly as among younger population groups and the elderly appear to have unique vulnerabilities to it. While the homeless are characterized by diversity among victims, clearly younger groups are characterized by some problems which are not so widely manifest among the elderly: visibility, diversity, minority, young, and single parents. Yet the housing problems of elderly Americans appear to go far beyond homelessness. Indeed, largely because of the shortage of available housing options, homelessness appears to represent only the tip of the iceberg of problems facing a significant proportion of elders who are poor, alone, and have been aging "in place" during the 1980s.

As many among the homeless appear to be experiencing a relatively new phenomenon, little is known about the elderly "new homeless." Knowledge is fragmented as each American city "discovers" homelessness on its own and documents its unique local manifestations. Studies are constrained by the very social construction of the term "homelessness" which suggests a dichotomous condition one has or does not have (Berman, Iris, Keigher, under review). Studies are further constrained by traditional ways of viewing the underclass, and by the wide variance in local history, development, and demographics in this country. The wide range of circumstances and housing problems which can capture elderly persons in the web of homelessness are difficult to analyze comprehensively. Many forces are relatively new and poorly documented.

The growth of homelessness appears to be related to the general housing problems of elderly in several ways. The poor elderly are caught in a growing shortage of low-income housing. In the past decade, gentrification, demolitions, federal program cutbacks, changing tax benefits, pre-payments and buy-outs of federal mortgages on rent-subsidized buildings have created a housing shortfall for the poor elderly in urban areas. This problem is expected to worsen in the next few years because so little new construction is "in the pipeline" (National Housing Task Force, 1988). The low income elderly, a group particularly at risk because of health and other social vulnerabilities, will become caught increasingly in this shortfall.

THE INCOME AND HOUSING PROBLEMS OF THE ELDERLY

Although a good deal of attention has been focused in recent years on the relative affluence of the elderly population, less attention has been paid to those segments of the elderly population most vulnerable to poverty. As a result of the Great Society initiatives over the last 30 years and especially with the indexing of Social Security in the early 1970s, the rate of poverty for the elderly is now less than that for the population as a whole. By 1988, the proportion of persons 65 years or older below the poverty level was 12%, compared with 25.3% in 1969 (Employee Benefit Research Institute, 1989). Despite such improvements, variables such as ethnicity, gender, and household type continue to have a significant impact on the likelihood of an elderly person living in poverty. According to the U.S. census, elderly blacks are more than three times as likely as elderly whites to have incomes below the poverty level, and elderly of Hispanic origin are more than twice as likely as elderly whites to be poor (U.S. Department of Commerce, 1990). Elderly females are twice as likely as elderly males to live in poverty; 12.6% of elderly females lived in poverty in 1987 compared with 6.1% of elderly males (U.S. Bureau of the Census, 1988). Household size is also a critical factor in poverty: 43% of the elderly living alone are poor or near poor, a rate nearly five times that of elderly couples and equal to the poverty rate of children (Commonwealth Fund, 1988).

The meager resources that poor elderly have to meet housing costs is compounded by the fact that such persons typically pay a much larger proportion of their income on housing related expenses. Although three out of four elderly headed households own their own homes, home ownership does not necessarily prevent housing related difficulties. According to recent reports, two out of three poor elderly homeowners spend at least 30% of their income on housing. Elderly renters, who comprise roughly one third of elderly households, are even more likely to face substantial housing costs. Three quarters of poor elderly renters spend at least 30% of their income on housing (U.S. Senate Special Committee on Aging, 1989, p. 275).

Elderly poor are also likely to experience housing related problems such as overpricing, substandard units, or crowded conditions. A recent Congressional Budget Office study found that 76% of very low income elderly renters experienced at least one of these three problems (Congressional Budget Office, 1988). Poor elderly are particularly vulnerable to a lack of social and physical supports which may become necessary as they age. This phenomenon, dubbed "Aging in Place" (American Association of Homes for the Aging, 1990) is of particular concern for owners of independent housing units for the elderly.

The growing proportion of elderly in the U.S. population over the next thirty years will necessitate increased attention to housing related problems. From 1980 to 1985, the percentage of households headed by persons over 65 has grown by 33%, and those headed by persons over 75 has increased by 52% (U.S. Senate Select committee on Aging, 1989). At the same time, the number of elderly in the population most vulnerable to poverty—ethnic minorities, women, and persons living alone—has grown at an even greater rate than the rest of the elderly population. Rising housing costs, deteriorating housing conditions, and the need for housing related support services for the elderly are problems which will demand immediate substantial attention as the United States moves toward the 21st century.

ERODING FEDERAL COMMITMENT TO AFFORDABLE HOUSING

At the same time as the number of elders has begun a noticeable growth, the nation's infrastructure of housing resources has begun to disappear. Budget authority in the assisted housing category of the Department of Housing and Urban Development declined from $25 billion in FY 1981 to $8.9 billion in FY 1990—a reduction of

80% in real dollars (U.S. Senate Special Committee on Aging, 1990). This declining Federal commitment to housing construction and rehabilitation will have profound impacts on the nation's ability to meet elderly housing needs in the future. The growing problem of buyouts of federally subsidized mortgages, as well as provisions affecting subsidized housing under the 1986 Tax Reform, are two issues that have particular impacts on elderly renters.

The prepayment of federally subsidized mortgages by owners of low income housing is a critical factor in the erosion of existing housing stock. Contracts which provide mortgage interest payments and other subsidies for owners of low income housing allow owners to pre pay 40 year mortgages after 20 years, thus ending their obligation to serve low income tenants. The prepayment problem affects residents living in a variety of privately owned housing projects, including those financed by Section 236 and 221(d) as well as projects financed with mortgage revenue bonds of which 20% of units are set aside for low and moderate income people. The American Association of Retired Persons estimates that 7-10% of federal housing for the elderly could be lost by prepayments during the 1990's (U.S. Senate Select Committee on Aging, 1989).

The 1986 Tax Reform Act included a number of provisions which have had the net effect of reducing the availability of rental housing for the elderly. These included a less generous depreciation schedule and limitations on the amount of rental loss that can be deducted by an investor. New restrictions require owners to set aside 40% of units for persons with less than 60% of median income. Although beneficial to renters who might not otherwise obtain housing, in practice this requirement has made it difficult for owners to obtain bond financing, particularly in urban areas with high housing costs. Uncertain tax incentives, combined with favorable private housing markets, have made conversion to private units particularly appealing (U.S. Senate Special Committee on Aging, 1989).

Although many concerned with Federal housing programs were hopeful that the start of the Bush administration would signal a reversal of the massive erosion of federal housing funding during the 1980's, in reality these hopes have not materialized. Instead, Federal attention in recent years has focused on the Federal budget deficit, publicity surrounding the H.U.D. scandals in the 1980's, and problems related to the drug infestation of public housing projects. Although the Housing and Community Development Acts of 1987 and 1989 address some of the problems related to the erosion of housing stock, the main thrust of these laws have been to address the serious management problems evident in H.U.D. in the 1980's and to provide oversight mechanisms to prevent further abuse. The many provisions within the Affordable Housing Act of 1990 (SB 566) appear to be a start toward addressing these issues, but a comprehensive strategy for redressing the erosion of Federal housing stock is unlikely to materialize in the present political environment. These concerns are manifest in the current status of several specific federal housing programs of particular interest to elderly Americans: those supporting traditional public housing, new construction, and vouchers or income enhancement.

Public Housing

Public housing represents the traditional and oldest form of housing assistance for the elderly. Approximately 45% of the nation's 1.2 million public housing units are occupied by older Americans. The deteriorating condition of public housing units, as well as the dangers posed by drug traffic, however, pose considerable problems for the elderly population in these units. Because only 50% of public housing units report any information on the functional levels of their residents, the Senate Special Committee on Aging (1989) reported that it is difficult to even estimate the extent of the problems that elderly face in public housing. It is likely that an increasing number of elderly are wary of living in such units, further decreasing their housing options and increasing the likelihood of homelessness. Finally, against the backdrop of housing stock erosion, H.U.D.'s own reputation for fraud and mismanagement has further eroded public confidence.

The current Administration's emphasis on privatization of public housing units represents a further threat to the supply of public housing stock. The Presidents' commission of privatization has recommended that public housing units be made available for sale to tenants or private investors. It has been suggested that the sale of these units, although helpful for some troubled projects, will result in a loss of operating subsidies and increase the likelihood of conversion of public housing units for new uses (Hearing on Select Committee on Aging, 1988).

The HUD Section 8 Program

The New Construction Program

Until 1983, the Department of Housing and Urban Development contracted with developers and builders for a specified number of units to be built to meet the needs of low income persons meeting federal eligibility standards for housing assistance. Under the Housing Act of 1983, the construction program, with the exception of units attached to the Sction 202 program, was repealed. Despite the termination of construction, existing Section 8 buildings continue to be an important source for the elderly: as of 1989, it was estimated that 48% of the 2.4 million Section 8 eligible units were occupied by older persons (Senate Special Committee on Aging, 1989).

The expiration of Section 8 contracts poses a serious threat to the provision of low income housing for the elderly. Because most Section 8 contracts were funded for 15 year terms during the years 1975 to 1980, as many as 200,000 to 300,000 units are due to expire between 1991 and 1994 (National Low Income Housing Information Service, 1990) Further housing erosion is expected as the result of building owners choosing to "opt out" of Section 8 contracts. Contracts signed before 1980 allow owners to get out of the Section 8 program at five year intervals. Opt outs are particularly attractive in urban areas with rapidly appreciating real estate costs. As a result, urban elderly are vulnerable to displacement as owners turn subsidized units into market rate rentals and condominiums (National Low Income Housing Information Service, 1990).

Section 8 Existing Housing Funding

The current section 8 existing housing program provides subsidies to help low income families and individuals meet housing costs. Under the Section 8 certificate program, H.U.D. pays the difference between units' actual rent and 30% of a tenants adjusted income. Eligible households may rent any existing unit that meets certain property standards and whose rent does not exceed the Fair Market Rent for a given area. The section 8 voucher program is similar to the certificate program, the major difference being that under the voucher program the dollar amount of the rental subsidy is fixed, and a family is free to rent a unit that may be above or below the 30% of income level. Started under an experimental basis in 1983, housing vouchers have become an increasingly prevalent means of providing low income housing. Funding for the voucher program in FY 1989 included $1,276 million for 47,000 new units, compared with $542 million for 18,000 new units under the certificate program (Congressional Budget Office, 1988). Although in theory housing vouchers give tenants greater options in the housing market, they also increase the likelihood that low income tenants will pay more than 30% of income for rent, particularly in high cost urban areas. As a result, even those poor elderly households receiving government housing assistance are likely to spend a large proportion of income on housing costs.

The Section 202 Program

The section 202 program for the elderly and handicapped is currently the primary program for the construction of housing for the elderly and handicapped, and is currently the only new construction program sponsored by H.U.D. Budget authority for Section 202 units has decreased by 81% since 1981. For 1991, the Bush Administration proposed reducing the number of new 202 units from less than 8,500 in FY 1990 to 3,967—a 53% reduction (U.S. Senate Special Committee on Aging, 1989, p. 387). Cost containment requirement within the Section 202 program, established by H.U.D. in 1981, represent a further reduction in services. The establishment of space limitations in individual units, limitations on congregate areas, and requirements that at least 25% of units be one room efficiencies are particularly detrimental to an increasingly frail elderly resident population. A survey of Section 202 managers found that only 14.2% of residents were completely independent in functioning in 1988, compared with 54% in 1983 (U.S. Senate Select Committee on Aging, 1989).

The shortage of Section 202 housing is a growing phenomenon, particularly in urban areas. An average of six Section 8 units are available for every 1,000 elderly persons in the U.S., and 1987 data shows a turnover rate of only 13.4%. In cities of more than 1 million persons, there are more than 11 applicants for every vacant 202 unit, a number that does not reflect the numbers of poor elderly who may be discouraged from even applying to the program due to the scarcity of 202 housing.

Single Room Occupancy (SRO) Housing

Since the turn of the century, Single Room Occupancy Hotels (SRO's) have been an important source of housing for low income inner city single residents. For single elderly with few personal or economic resources, SRO hotels have been outstanding among the few alternatives available. Despite recognition of the value of this form of private market housing, the outlook for financing of such housing looks particularly bleak. The Bush 1991 budget proposes a cut of almost one third in the Section 8 moderate rehabilitation program which would assist such hotels. The $49.6 million requested for rental assistance would provide for only 1,305 rooms nationwide. These units, previously available to all homeless persons, would be integrated into the Shelter Plus Care program and as a result be limited to mentally ill persons or recovering substance abusers. Elderly who are not classified in these two categories would be prohibited from obtaining housing in the small number of SRO units which would be made available (National Low Income Housing Information Service, 1990). Although SROs are likely to remain as an option for persons able to pay private market rates, eroding federal commitment will contribute to the destruction and elimination of many units.

HOMELESSNESS AND THE AGING POPULATION

Homelessness Programs

As a result of the increased attention paid to homelessness by the media and various advocacy groups during the 1980s, the federal government has shown interest in targeting particularly visible and apparently vulnerable populations, including the elderly, for limited special assistance. This has been most true of the McKinney Act. The Stewart B. McKinney Act, signed into law on July 22, 1987, is the Federal governments' major provision to assist local governments and agencies in providing services for the homeless. The program includes funding programs within a number of governmental units including the Department of Housing and Urban Development, Department of Health and Human Services, and the Departments of Labor, Education, and Agriculture (U.S. Senate Select Committee on Aging, 1989). Most increases for the 1991 budget were proposed in the category of rental housing assistance for the homeless, a program which is the centerpiece of the Bush HOPE plan (Housing Opportunities for People Everywhere). The Rental Housing Assistance plan, which was not part of the original McKinney legislation, would provide rental assistance and other support services for homeless persons with mental illness or chronic alcohol problems. Because this program replaces the Supplemental Assistance for Facilities to Assist the Homeless (SAFAH) program, which provided comprehensive strategies for all homeless persons, the Rental Housing Assistance Program basically represents an abandonment of a previously existing program serving the elderly homeless (National Low Income Housing Information Service, 1990).

In short, the Administration's efforts of the last decade have been of symbolic importance at best, and at worst an effective comprehensive strategy to abandon any federal role in public provision of housing altogether. The prospects for federal maintenance of support for low income housing for elders, much less for the creation of new housing resources to meet needs of a rapidly aging population, are bleak at best. The stage is set, given the current indicators and projections, for a crisis of unprecedented magnitude as we look at the emergent issues and human costs.

A recent Institute of Medicine study found in a review of 13 studies in 8 cities, that persons over age 60 comprise anywhere from 2.5 to 9% of the homeless, while they are 15.6% of the general population (Institute of Medicine, 1988). This apparent underrepresentation of the aged among the homeless may be due to their eligibility at age 65 to a number of public benefits (Social Security,

Medicare, senior housing, etc.) which generates enough income to facilitate their leaving the streets or prevents them from becoming homeless in the first place. The debilitating circumstances in which the homeless live suggest that a lower number of homeless individuals survive to old age. It is also possible that this proportion merely reflects the sampling methodology of the studies, since most study subjects are self selected and include shelter residents or persons already seeking services and thus exclude persons living in the streets. It is also likely that the elderly are less prone to use such services. It is widely acknowledged that shelters are dangerous places and that younger homeless persons tend to "squeeze out" older ones (Institute of Medicine, 1988, p. 16).

THE IMPACTS OF HOUSING EROSION ON THE ELDERLY OF CHICAGO

The erosion of federal commitment to housing has been compounded in Chicago by a reduction in the availability of private low-cost housing. The cumulative effect raises the spectre of housing hardships among a wide cross-section of low income populations, hardships that can be felt and seen in raw human terms in the faces of the homeless in most cities. It certainly raised for us concerns about how some elders in the community were being affected by the late 1980's and what could be done about it.

The majority of this special issue examines a sample of older Chicagoans who have experienced a serious emergency that brought them to the attention of city agencies. Drawn from city agency client data files, the sampled clients' needs and service patterns provide insight into the nature of problems major cities are facing. The data reveal some important correlates of housing related crises and unmet need for temporary shelter.

An Aging Population Amidst Urban Constraints

Like cities throughout the country, Chicago has seen an unprecedented growth in the elderly population, an increase which is especially pronounced among the oldest elderly. People over age 60 represent an ever larger proportion of the city's population, and those over age 85, who are the most vulnerable to loss of familial support, income, and health, are the fastest growing subgroup among the elderly (U.S. Census, 1982). The population of older blacks and other minorities is growing just as rapidly, and the proportion of blacks over age 85 is growing even more rapidly than for other racial groups (Kingson, Hirshorn, & Cornman, 1986; Squires, Bennett, McCourt & Nyden, 1988).

Ethnic sensitivity in housing is high in Chicago, a city notorious historically for its segregated neighborhoods. The Department of Aging and Disability recently identified at least fifty distinct ethnic groups among the elderly. Dislocated individuals and families are often limited to relocating near family and within certain ethnic boundaries. Ethnic traditions of family care and availability of non-employed potential caregivers vary greatly. Ethnicity of particular neighborhoods contributes to locally unique needs, housing stock, and community demands. The supply of decent housing in the oldest and most deteriorated neighborhoods and of low income housing in neighborhoods which are gentrifying cannot keep up with the demand. Many families are not available or able to care for and support their elderly relatives. Although poor persons may be able to reside at least temporarily with their families, such arrangements contribute to crowded conditions. Ironically, families with the poorest incomes frequently have time and commitment to help out but have little space or economic resources to offer.

City Services for the Elderly

City agencies are not equipped to intervene substantially with older persons who do not ask for help, who have no family, or who do not go to senior centers and congregate meal sites. Yet, increasingly these persons—who tend to be very old, poor, and living alone (Butler, 1975; Butler and Davis, 1986)—are in need of multiple services. Support for client autonomy and the right to be left alone is often raised as a justification for the state's complex and rather weak provisions for guardianship. Agencies are discouraged from intervening aggressively with even desperately ill and demented older clients who are perceived as uncooperative, at least partially because they lack legal backup and sufficient alternative housing resources.

Growth has been gradual but greatest among particular segments of the elderly population, the very old, poor and persons living alone, persons who appear to be the most reluctant or least able to use traditional city services. Growth of these groups appears to have contributed to increased demands on city emergency services. Emergency service referrals of older persons increased dramatically in 1986 and 1987 (Keigher, 1987). The shelter system in Chicago, which the city human service agency supports and which is relatively extensive and well developed, operates at more than full capacity between November and April, serving approximately 1 in 10 of the homeless by the city's estimates. But the city emergency service agency does not meet the needs of the general homeless population, much less serve the special needs of the elderly. It has tried to involve the city agency on aging in providing more services to its elderly clients, but given their limited resources, city agencies serving seniors must evaluate how and to what extent to respond.

Adding to this pressure is the fact that the number of nursing home and psychiatric hospital beds to which mentally ill older people might be committed are limited and not likely to increase. The Illinois Department of Mental Health substantially reduced the number of custodial and treatment beds in state institutions over the last twenty years and the state Department on Aging instituted nursing home preadmission screening in 1982. With Medicaid support, it began funding home and community based services – home care, chore, and housekeeping services. Yet, these services were not designed to care for persons in emergencies who are either homeless, seriously confused, uncooperative, or otherwise unwilling to accept assistance. The aging network, like most social services, appears to respond more deliberately and decisively to abuse and neglected elderly persons than to those suffering from "self-neglect" or in need of decent housing. The city's capacity to respond to broad social problems is seriously constrained.

Loss of Affordable Housing Stock

The last, and probably most important trend, is that Chicago, like the rest of the nation, is losing the housing units which low-income individuals can afford (U.S. Department of Commerce Annual Housing Survey, 1985), gradually imposing systemic stress on poor and marginally functioning people. Units are being lost in both the market economy and in subsidized developments. Chicago has experienced a precipitous loss of Single Room Occupancy (SRO) and other low-income housing stock in recent years due to condominium conversion, gentrification, and razing by private developers as well as by the city itself. Hoch (1985) notes that 1,000 SRO units are being lost each year, and if that trend continues, SROs in Chicago will completely disappear by about 1995. The City Department of Planning (December 1987, p. iv) notes that between 1973 and 1984, approximately 18,000 units of housing in SROs and other low-income structures with small dwelling units were removed from the housing supply.

During this same period some 17,000 units of subsidized senior housing was added to the city supply, and the population living in nursing homes increased from 24,202 in 1970 to 37,573 in 1980. These publicly subsidized structures absorbed much of the growth in the elderly population during the 1970s, even as the supply of market available stock stagnated (City of Chicago, Department of Planning, 1987, p. 34).

As a result of this erosion, very old people who are poor and who live alone present a distinct challenge to agencies trying to manage their problems. Because of these trends, Chicago officials expect to see increasing homelessness among the elderly in the next few years. Among other things, alleviation of homelessness and housing problems will require a better understanding of their victims.

The Extent of Homelessness in Chicago

The Chicago Coalition on the Homeless estimated there were 25,000 homeless persons of all ages in Chicago in 1983, and the Chicago Task Force on Emergency Shelter that same year estimated there were 12,000 to 25,000 such persons (p.2). Peter Rossi's Chicago study (1987) estimated that in the winter of 1986 there were only 4-6,000 homeless persons at any one time. The widely varying estimates suggest that counting the homeless has become highly politicized. Estimating the proportion of the homeless who are a given age is similarly tricky. Rossi noted that 19.4% of those living on the streets were over age 55. The City Department of Human Services records indicate that in 1987 there were 6,000 regular shelter users, of whom only about 6% were over age 55. The disparity among these proportions may indicate that the elderly are a greater share of those on the streets than those staying in shelters. A recent Institute of Medicine study (1988) indicates that the elderly have good reasons to fear shelters which they perceive as dangerous places (pp. 15-17). It seems very likely that a greater proportion of the elderly are in need than are receiving assistance in shelters.

Several other studies of homelessness (Sosin, 1987, 1988; Hasleberger, 1987; Hannibal, 1984) indicate that older persons in Chicago are suffering the increase in homelessness at least as much as younger populations. Their difficulties appear to be less with finding housing (as is the case with young families) than with keeping and maintaining their homes independently. Declining physical mobility makes their plight less visible, and their higher rate of home ownership often masks the true proportions of chronically marginal living conditions. While the general economic status of the elderly has steadily improved throughout the 1970s and 1980s, the poor among the elderly appear to be worse off than ever. This has important implications as we consider the kind of interventions that will truly prevent housing loss among the elderly.

Recent studies in Chicago (Rossi, 1986; Kutza, 1987; and Sosin, Colson & Grossman, 1988) and Detroit (Douglass, 1988) present a somewhat inconsistent picture of the urban elderly homeless. Street surveys suggest that they are largely men (Rossi), while samples from agencies serving elderly homeless clients are largely women (Kutza). Street surveys find the homeless elderly to be relatively young, between 55 and 65 (Douglass, 1988), while Kutza's agency data found the homeless to be quite old. Rossi found the "elderly" (age 55 and over) to be 19% of the homeless on the street and Sosin found them to be 12% of persons in his study at meal and shelter programs, while the city's population age 55 and over is 21.2% (1980 U.S. Census for City of Chicago). So even in this city with a relatively high proportion of elderly among the homeless, they are proportionately under-represented. Elderly blacks are somewhat over-represented in all of these studies.

Monthly reports of the Chicago Department of Human Service (DHS) reveal an increasing elderly caseload. Between January 1986 and August 1987 the agency experienced a 400% increase in referrals of elders from its emergency service unit to its senior followup unit. Categorizing only the primary presenting problems, 59% of all cases identified the reason for referral as basic needs, including: need for shelter or temporary housing, deteriorated or deplorable housing conditions, fire, eviction, tenant-landlord disputes, and others. Twenty-nine percent of the cases present medical needs, 4% involve victimization, and 9% involve a wide variety of other problems. The nature of these cases has not changed much as they increased, although the proportion involving fires, need for shelter and need for medical care appear to have increased somewhat, and housing and medical problems continued to be the most prevalent emergencies. (The "need for food" has all but disappeared, however, since the agency stopped issuing emergency food boxes after March 1987.)

In order to examine these needs more closely, and to see how they fit into the larger context of a shrinking supply of affordable housing, our study, reported in the next two chapters, analyzes a large random sample of seniors who have had emergencies. In the process it explores the "bounded nature" of agency generated data as valid indicators of need. Cases drawn from the agency's emergency files shed light on: the characteristics of the elderly in Chicago who come to the attention of the city; the extent of their housing related need; and why some elderly use city shelters and how their problems precipitate shelter use. These clients have a broad range of putative needs and some are at particularly high risk of losing their housing. To identify factors associated with persons who have been homeless, it compares those who have needed shelter with those who have not, providing a tentative glimpse of the patterns to housing loss and risk experienced by the elderly in the late 1980s.

REFERENCES

American Association of Homes for the Aging. (1990). *Aging in place: Supporting the frail elderly in residential environments*. Glenview, IL: Scott, Foresman and Company.

Berman, R., Iris, M., & Keigher, S. (under review). The Continuum of Homelessness. *Housing and Society*.

Butler, R. (1975). *Why survive? Being old in America*. New York: Harper.

Butler, R. & Davis, K. (1986) *Old, alone and poor: A plan for reducing poverty among elderly people living alone*. New York: The Commonwealth Fund Commission.

City of Chicago, Department of Planning (1987, Dec.)

Commonwealth Fund Commission on Elderly Living Alone. (1988). *Aging alone: Profiles and Projections*. Baltimore, MD: Author.

Congressional Budget Office. (1988). *Current housing problems and possible federal response* (No. 92-492 0-89-1). Washington, D.C.: U.S. Government Printing Office.

Douglass, R. (1988). *Aged, alone and adrift*. Detroit Area Agency on Aging.

Employee Benefit Research Institute. (1989). The economic well-being of the elderly: Past, present, and future. *Employee Benefit Research Institute Issue Brief*, *96*, 1-17.

Hannibal, C. (1984, March). *Out of the mainstream and into the streets: A preliminary study of homeless women in the Chicago Loop*. Chicago: Community Emergency Shelter Organization.

Haslberger, A. (1987). *Homelessness in New Town*. Chicago: Community Emergency Shelter Organization.

Hoch, C. (1985). *SROs: An endangered species*. Chicago: Community Emergency Shelter Organization and Jewish Council on Urban Affairs.

Institute of Medicine. (1988). *Homelessness, health, and human needs*. Washington, D.C.: National Academy Press.

Keigher, S. (1987). *The city's responsibility for the homeless elderly of Chicago*. Gerontological Society of America Fellowship Report: Chicago Department of Aging and Disability.

Kingson, E., Hirshorn, B. & Cornman, J. *Ties that bind*. The Gerontological Society of America: Washington, DC.

Kutza, E. (1987). *Undomiciled elderly persons in Chicago*. Park Ridge, IL: Retirement Research Foundation.

National coalition of the Homeless. (undated). *Homelessness in America: A summary*. New York.

National Low Income Housing Information Service. (1990). Expiring section 8 contracts: Renewing the promise of affordable housing (Order #SM-190). Washington, D.C.: Author.

National Housing Task Force. (1988, March). *A decent place to live*. Washington, DC.

National Low Income Housing Information Service. (1990). *The fiscal year 1991 budget and low income housing* (#SM-290). Washington, D.C.

Rossi, P., Fisher, G. & Willis, G. (1986). *The condition of the homeless of Chicago*. Chicago: National Opinion Research Center.

Sosin, M., Colson, P. & Grossman, S. (1988, June). *Homelessness in Chicago*. Chicago: School of Social Service Administration, The University of Chicago and Chicago Community Trust.

Squires, G.D., Bennett, L., McCourt, K. & Nyden, P. (1988). *Chicago: Race, class and the response to urban decline*. Philadelphia: Temple University Press.

U.S. National Conference of Mayors. (1986, June). *Responding to homelessness in America's cities*. Washington, DC: U.S. Conference of Mayors.

U.S. Senate Select Committee on Aging, (1989). *The 1988 national survey of section 202 housing for the elderly and handicapped* (Committee Publication 101-736). Washington, D.C.:U.S. Government Printing Office.

U.S. Senate. Special Committee on Aging, (1990). *Developments in Aging: 1989* (Report No. 101-249). Washington, D.C.: U.S. Government Printing Office.

U.S. Department of Commerce, Bureau of the Census. (1985). *Annual Housing Survey*.

U.S. Department of Commerce, Bureau of the Census. (1990). *Statistical Abstract of the United States* (110th ed.). Washington, D.C.: Author.

U.S. Department of Commerce, Bureau of the Census. (1982). *Chicago*.

Chapter 2

Overview of the Chicago Study of Elderly Persons at Housing Risk

Sharon M. Keigher
Rebecca Hanson Berman
Sadelle T. Greenblatt

SUMMARY. This chapter presents the basic approach and research design of the Chicago study which was directed at studying homelessness as one of many housing risks of the elderly. Both quantitative and qualitative methods of analysis utilized are described here, while a more detailed explanation of the process can be found in the Appendix. Data sources, sample selection methods, and data collection procedures are described, as well as the approach, methods and statistical tests used in the comparative analysis.

According to city agencies in Chicago (the departments on aging, human services, fire and police), poverty, desperate housing problems, and near-homelessness are prevalent among identifiable subgroups of the elderly. The Chicago Department of Human Services (DHS), the city agency charged with providing emergency shelter and services on a 24 hour basis, paid for shelter for 600 different persons aged 60 and over in 1987. Nearly a third of the 82,000 emergency calls to its Emergency Services program in the first eight months of 1988 were housing-related, as were over half of those to which the department sent out an emergency response team. Such housing emergencies included evictions, need for shelter, "deplorable housing conditions," fires, assaults and other destruction that led to dislocation, tenant landlord disputes, utility shutoffs, and be-

The authors acknowledge the advice and consultation provided by Madelyn Iris in the construction of the research design and approach to the coding, management and analysis of the qualitative data.

ing chronically undomiciled. A substantial proportion of these emergencies suggest the presence of other social problems that could precipitate homelessness, and many appear to be preventable.

Indeed, according to DHS staff, housing related emergencies appear to be even more common proportionately among older persons (aged 60 and over) than among younger persons served by DHS. Keigher (1987) found that at least half of these emergencies experienced by the elderly were housing related. Older poor persons who live alone and have no family ties are widely recognized for being at especially high risk (Butler and Davis, 1986).

The extent to which such problems lead to homelessness and institutionalization, however, is unknown. Keigher's study suggested that among the elderly, near-homelessness (deplorable housing conditions, fires, and having to relocate) may be as threatening to health, safety, and life itself as is the experience of having no place to live. Persons in an emergency appear to be at a critical juncture which often leads to relocation. How they cope and the options available to them are important determinants of what happens next and whether further dislocation and trauma is prevented. We need to know more about who is truly at risk and their options.

Alternatives in such emergencies, aside from those offered by relatives and friends, depend largely upon the availability of appropriate housing, but since the supply is often inadequate, DHS Emergency Services often use paid shelter, motels, and nursing homes along with free shelters. In contrast to this, single room occupancy (SRO) hotels are one of the most affordable and flexible types of housing for inner-city poor people, although the stock of SRO housing in Chicago, as in other places, is limited and rapidly shrinking. In the gerontological literature, SROs have been widely acknowledged as socially supportive, convenient, and reasonably priced alternative housing for seniors. While often inadequately recognized as a resource, SROs sustain important informal helping networks and have been widely utilized by governments in time of necessity because of their convenience. Today the reduced supply of SROs is playing an increasingly important role to cities facing housing shortages and to all levels of government looking for market mechanisms to solve their problems. Given the current importance of low-income housing, a better understanding of the value of SRO housing to the poor elderly who remain independent—persons who are not asking for nor using services—can be especially useful.

PURPOSE

The study presented in most of this volume describes the characteristics and housing patterns of older persons in Chicago who have experienced homelessness and other serious housing problems. It compares a sample of seniors with housing problems with another sample living in SROs who are, presumably, coping more successfully, comparing their needs and resources, both internal and external. From these two populations, those selected because they had been served by ES and problems and a comparison group in a similar socioeconomic position, who have not been served by ES, we can learn also about successful coping. This can provide insight into factors that act as barriers to homelessness among the elderly and ways SROs might be improved and strengthened as a housing option for the elderly on very limited incomes.

METHODOLOGY

The first portion of the study examines clients of the Emergency Services Division of the Chicago Department of Human Services, and other individuals who are currently living in SROs—two groups of elders who are living independently in the community, one who have had crises and one who have not. The second part (reported in Part III of this volume along with a national SRO study by Ovrebo, Minkler and Liljestrand) examines a sample of Chicago SRO hotels themselves, their populations, their amenities, and the supports they provide for their residents. Below is a brief discussion of our methods of sample selection, data collection process, and analysis. A more detailed discussion of methodology can be found in the Appendix of this volume.

The Client Study

The client study includes two groups of individuals – those identified from the records of the Emergency Services Division of the Chicago Department of Human Services (ES) and those identified in our survey of SROs. Based on analysis of a large random sample of ES clients we identified two groups of housing related problems which appear to place clients at "housing risk" especially for relocation. We selected a sample of ES clients who (1) "have needed shelter" and (2) have experienced other housing related problems. These clients are compared with a third group, (persons expected to be similar demographically) (3) persons living in single room occupancy hotels. The SRO residents were selected from hotels throughout the city in order to more clearly see their residential histories and associated problems.

Random sampling of the Emergency Services clients indicates that persons over age 60 represent approximately 11% of all names in the ES case files. A random sample of 475 elderly individuals was drawn from the contact cards in these files (see Appendix for a more detailed explanation). These client cards include cases for which the most recent contact occurred up to four years ago, allowing case histories to be constructed retrospectively. Although ES does not do case management, another DHS unit, the Division of Youth and Family Services (YFS) Senior Unit, does provide follow-up.

Data from these 475 randomly selected records were collected and the presenting problems identified. Using these data, a "housing risk" sub-set was identified consisting of 129 clients who at last contact with ES had (a) needed temporary housing or shelter, or (b) were in deplorable housing conditions. Comparison of the demographic characteristics of the random sample and this sub-set indicates that there are no statistically significant differences between the two groups. From this housing risk sub-set and another random sample selected in a pilot study, a purposive sample of 115 cases (126 persons) were selected for investigation and interview. In the SRO sub-sample thirty individuals living in the surveyed SROs were randomly selected and interviewed. The same interview instrument was used in assessing both samples.

In addition to the respondent interviews, the process of data collection for the housing risk interview sample of ES clients involved also gathering data from the YFS records on any contacts with that division of the agency. Information collected from the ES and YFS records includes client demographics, presenting problems, services needed, services provided, date and number of agency contacts, names of other individuals or agencies involved with the clients, and the client's last known address.

From July through November 1988, researchers attempted to locate the selected housing risk clients, contacting all residences, agencies, friends, and relatives that could be identified from the agency records. In-person qualitative interviews were conducted with located respondents and informants for both groups in the subsample. An assessment was made using an augmented OARS instrument (more fully described in the Appendix) covering health and mental status, functional capacity, social support,and economic resources. Exploratory discussion about the chronology of housing problems and relocations secured a housing history and identified critical combinations of factors that appeared to have precipitated emergency situations.

The Study of SROs

This study builds upon the findings from a 1985 Chicago study by Charles Hoch, *SROs: An Endangered Species*. Our objectives were to update our understanding of the value of SROs, to identify critical features of social and economic life in SROs that could be strengthened to improve residents' access to needed services, and to identify residents' options and preferences should hotels in three specific threatened locales actually be lost.

First a representative sample of hotels was selected. All of the 18 hotels in Hoch's 1985 study (which were a stratified representative sample) were included in our sample. Additional hotels were selected according to the following criteria: (1) average rent was below $220 according to the 1985 data; (2) the hotel appeared to have a significant number or proportion of older residents; and (3) a contact person willing to talk could be located on site. The total sample was to include (4) hotels of varying size; and (5) each area in the city which has a concentration of low-rent SROs. All areas represented in the ES client sample were included as much as feasible. Using these criteria, a total of 15 additional hotels were selected.

Actual data collection involved the following. A survey and interviews with hotel staff and with the residents who form the SRO client sample were conducted at 27 hotels, including 12 of the original 18 hotels and the 15 additional selections. In addition to the interviews with residents, short questionnaires were completed with about 40 other older residents.

Statistical Tests and Methodological Limitations

In the data analysis reported in Chapters 3 and 7, the statistical tests used were difference of proportions, difference of means, and chi square. For all tests, the level of significance was set at the .05 level.

Because of the very short-term contact by ES staff with clients in emergency situations, much of the data are missing for the clients who could not be located during the study. While there were no statistically significant differences between the ES client sample and the 115 in the sub-sample selected for interview, it was not possible to locate 23% of the individuals selected for the interview sample, despite the extensive search we describe later. Even the minimal data available, however, suggests these missing clients do have many characteristics which are salient to homelessness.

In comparing the sub-sample actually located (on whom we have a great deal of data, including interviews) with the random sample, the located interview sample are characterized by having more problems noted in the record and more referrals to Emergency Services. Though the whole of the interviewed sample shows no significant demographic difference from the random sample, we cannot conclude that no difference exists, since much of the these data were missing for the not located part of the sample. Therefore, while their experiences were highly informative, the interviewed sample are not necessarily representative of all ES elderly clients.

REFERENCES

Butler, R. N. & Davis, K. (1986). *Old, poor and alone*. New York: The Commonwealth Fund.

Hoch, C. (1985). *SRO's: an endangered species*. Chicago: Community Emergency Shelter Organization and Jewish Council on Urban Affairs.

Keigher, S. (1987). *The city's responsibility for the homeless elderly*. Chicago Department of Aging and Disability.

PART II: THE HOMELESS AND NEAR-HOMELESS ELDERLY AND HOW THEY COPE

Chapter 3

Older Emergency Service Clients and SRO Residents: Characteristics, Problems and Needs

Sharon M. Keigher
Sadelle T. Greenblatt

SUMMARY. A sample of 126 "housing risk" clients were identified for interview from agency emergency service cases. Records provided some history on the persistence of client need and were supplemented by in-person interviews with clients and ancillary informants. Ninety-one clients were located and their situations were compared with those of 30 randomly selected SRO residents. Comparison of these samples show that particular vulnerability to homelessness exists among those whose resources are impaired.

In this chapter, data from DHS agency records are used to describe the characteristics of a random sample of 475 aged ES clients who might be vulnerable to housing problems, and to identify and then compare two housing risk sub-groups using the agency's own problem categories as descriptive variables: those who at most recent contact had needed emergency shelter or temporary housing, and those who had been living in "deplorable housing conditions." (The latter usually means conditions ranging from unsafe or uninhabitable to having no utilities.) Following this, detailed information on client needs and services was gathered through interviews with the sub-sample of housing related cases we were able to locate. Then the three groups interviewed, the ES shelter clients, the ES poor housing clients, and the SRO clients, are compared. Our purpose here is to be statistically descriptive and to identify significant risk factors. The significant findings are summarized at the end of this chapter for readers who may not require this level of detail.

CHARACTERISTICS OF EMERGENCY SERVICE CLIENTS

Four-fifths of the older ES clients are living in their own apartments or homes, 11% are said to be living "on the streets" or in shelters, and 9% are scattered among SROs, nursing homes, and the homes of relatives (12% are unknown). Of those whose household composition is known, at least a third live alone, but household composition is unknown in 86% of the case records, and marital status is unknown in 91% of the cases.

Demographically ES clients are similar to the city's population age 60 and over, except that they are older and proportionately more black. Fifty-nine percent are female, as are 59% of the city's age 60 and over population. Forty-four percent are 75 or older, compared to only 26.5% for the city. Of those whose race is known, 45% are white as compared to 72% for the city as a whole (1980 census data). Thus ES clients aged 60 and over are more likely to be poor, because of their minority status, and disabled, because of their age. (See Table 3.1.)

Though the data on the location of the emergency are missing on 28% of the cases, the available data indicate that emergencies tend to occur unevenly across the city. Using police districts as identifiers, the Wentworth district (2) has the most senior emergency cases, followed by Englewood (7), Grand Crossing (3), and West

Table 3.1. Comparison of Random Sample to Chicago Elderly

Characteristic	Population age 60+ Chicago	Sample
proportion female	59.3%	59%
proportion white	71.7%	45%
proportion age 75 and older	26.7%	44%

Loop (12). Districts with the highest number of housing related cases are nearly the same, districts 2, 7, 23 (Uptown), 12 (Monroe), and 24 (Rogers Park). The incidence of housing related cases appear to be related to such factors as poor conditions of housing, scarcity of low rent units, the visibility of persons without homes, as well as long standing patterns of poverty and racial segregation. All of these conditions are particularly prevalent on the south and west sides. The need for shelter is particularly clustered in neighborhoods that have experienced urban renewal, but which used to have a high concentration of SROs and flop houses.

Analysis of the problems presented at the most recent ES contact reveals that about half of the clients present only one problem; but 29.1% present at least two and 7.6% present four or more. Certain housing related incidents, especially fires, rarely result in a second contact with ES, while multiple contacts often occur with certain types of problems, especially with problems such as need for emergency shelter, and clients presenting evidence of multiple problems.

A wide array of needs are revealed by the problems to which ES responds. The most frequently listed primary problems are fire, being lost or confused, needing transportation, and needing temporary housing. Analysis of only these primary problems shows that housing related incidents account for 47% of all contacts with ES, and a substantial proportion of the incidents involving "lost seniors" and the need for transportation (another 32% of contacts) also appear to be related to housing needs. This is especially true of clients who live alone or are homeless. Undoubtedly, due to the focus on the immediate resolution of the emergency, many problems are overlooked or minimized in the data drawn from the ES records. Yet, it is noteworthy that mental illness or alcoholism are recorded in only 11% of the cases in the ES sample.

Client records indicate that the service provided is truly the emergency assistance that it is designed to be, as the vast majority of clients are never seen again. For example, 78% of clients are seen only once, 10% are seen 3 or more times, and 3.8% are seen six or more times. About 86% of cases are resolved in less than one week, while nearly 9% are seen over a period longer than a month. It is this latter group, the repeaters, that have multiple and more complex problems.

Of the 475 cases in the random sample, shelter is mentioned in the record for 158 cases (33%), poor housing conditions for 59 (12%), fire for 97 (35%), eviction for 27 (6%), and need for temporary shelter for 96 (20%). As Table 3.2, below, indicates, there is considerably more overlap among the problems of persons who need shelter than with those of any of the other groups. Note how few needing shelter had also experienced fires. (Fires were usually the only problem noted.) Having had repeated referrals suggests that a substantial proportion of older persons who have needed shelter have had other serious needs requiring further help from ES. These are more clearly identified by examining how problems cluster and how they persist over time.

Of the 475 persons in the sample, 105 had been seen more than once. These clients present a clustering of problems at each contact. Certain problem combinations tend to have corollary needs and to produce certain outcomes. For example, transportation is a corollary need for 32% of the clients needing shelter; temporary shelter is

Table 3.2. Problems Occurring With Need for Shelter

Temporary housing and/or shelter	105
Temporary housing and/or shelter + fire	15
Temporary housing and/or shelter + eviction	15
Temporary housing and/or shelter + hsg. conds.	13
Temporary housing and/or shelter + fire + hsg conds	2
Needs shelter + fire + eviction	3
Needs shelter + fire + housing conditions	3
Needs shelter + housing conditions + eviction	2
Total	158

a corollary need for 19% of the wanderers and a resultant need for 33% of the evicted.

Some problems are particularly persistent, as they are listed at both the first and the last contact with ES. The persistence rate for "needs temporary shelter" is 68% and for poor housing conditions is 33%. Among the 54 cases in which either temporary shelter, shelter, or homelessness are mentioned, and which have multiple contacts with ES, the records indicate that in eight cases homelessness persisted for over a year. Most follow-up contacts occur rather quickly, especially with the group in need of shelter, but the high effort required to resolve the problems presented by such clients suggests the need to look more closely at them and how they differ from the other aged ES clients.

The Housing Problems of the ES Clients

The analysis described above identified four sub-groups for comparison: clients whose record with ES never mentions either poor housing conditions or need for shelter or temporary housing (A); those where shelter or temporary housing are mentioned (B1); those where poor housing conditions are mentioned (B2); and those where both of these problems are mentioned (B3). (See Table 3.3.)

Race is unknown in 36% of the cases, making findings on this characteristic somewhat inconclusive, but blacks appear to be overrepresented in all the housing risk groups (B1-B3) at 53 to 62% white, less white than the 72% white in the Chicago elderly population. The poor housing conditions group is the oldest, the most likely to be living in their own homes or apartments, the least likely to have been referred more than once, and the most likely to have been referred two or more years ago. There appear to be a declining number of housing conditions cases each year and of all ES problems, these were the most likely to also have utility shut-off problems. The group in need of temporary shelter has the highest proportion of men, the largest proportion that were living on the streets or in shelter, and the largest number that were referred within the past year. This group appears to be getting larger each year. The cases with both poor housing conditions and need for shelter have the highest proportion of women. They were the most likely to have

TABLE 3.3. Demographic Data for Sample Drawn in 1988

Sample*	Whole Sample	Type A	Type B1	Type B2	type B3
Characteristics	n=475	n=287	n=129	n=38	n=21
Modal age group	60-64	65-69	70-74	75-79	70-74
Sex (percent female)	58.5	60.4	53.2	60.5	61.9
Race (percent white)	44.7	37.9	53.3	57.7	50.0
Major source of last referral	CPD	CPD	CPD	CPD	CPD
Year of last referral					
% 1985	23.9	21.3	25.2	39.5	23.8
% 1986	27.7	30.3	22.8	28.9	19.0
% 1987	27.7	28.9	25.2	18.4	42.9
% 1988	20.7	19.5	26.8	13.2	14.3
Number of ES contacts					
1	77.8	85.0	64.3	78.9	61.9
2	12.0	10.5	17.1	10.5	4.8
3-5	6.3	3.1	10.9	7.9	19.1
6-10	3.2	1.3	5.5	2.6	14.3
11-15	0.0	0.0	0.0	0.0	0.0
over 15	0.6	0.0	2.4	0.0	0.0
Living arrangement at referral:					
Own home or apartment	79.8	88.5	51.2	94.7	76.2
Not known	12.2	9.4	22.5	2.6	0.0
Streets or shelter	10.6	1.2	29.8	2.6	14.3
SRO	3.8	3.8	4.0	0.0	4.8
Nursing Home	3.6	4.2	3.2	0.0	0.0
Relative's home	2.2	2.3	2.4	0.0	0.0
Primary problem at last referral:					
Fire	18.9	27.2	8.5	2.6	0.0
Wanderer/confused/lost	18.9	23.0	17.8	0.0	4.8
Needs Transportation	13.5	17.8	8.5	0.0	4.8
Needs temporary shelter	12.6	0.0	45.7	0.0	4.8
Other	11.7	14.6	7.0	5.2	14.4
Run down housing	6.7	0.0	0.0	57.9	47.6
Needs assessment of situation and needs	4.8	6.6	2.3	2.6	0.0
Victimization	3.2	4.5	1.6	0.0	0.0
Eviction	2.9	2.8	3.9	2.6	0.0
No utilities	2.9	0.0	0.0	26.3	19.0
Needs medical care or assessment	2.5	2.8	2.3	2.6	0.0
Needs other housing	.6	.3	1.6	0.0	0.0
Total number of problems:					
1	51.2	65.9	28.7	36.8	14.3
2	29.1	23.0	36.4	52.6	23.8
3	11.6	7.0	21.7	2.6	28.6
4	5.7	3.8	7.8	5.3	19.0
5 or more	1.9	0.0	3.9	2.6	14.3

*Type A cases had no record of need for temporary housing nor of poor housing conditions. Type B1 had a record of need for temporary housing but not of poor housing conditions. Type B2 had a record of poor housing conditions, but not of need for temporary housing. Type B3 had a record of both poor housing conditions and need for temporary housing.

multiple contacts with ES and multiple problems noted in the record. As was expected, the housing risks groups (Types B1-B3) had significantly higher rates of both total problems and number of referrals to ES. (See Table 3.3.)

THE HOUSING AND RELOCATION PROBLEMS OF INTERVIEWED ES CLIENTS AND SRO RESIDENTS

While the interviewed sample differs somewhat from the larger random sample and the housing risk subsample, it provides important basic information about the ES clients. Substantial difficulties were encountered in attempting to locate the housing risk clients selected for interview (see Appendix A), especially those who move frequently or have been without a home for long periods. The following analysis of the interview sample consists of the 91 ES clients aged 60 and over on whom complete data was gathered (including 37 with a history of poor housing conditions and 54 with a need for temporary housing or shelter) and 27 SRO residents aged 60 and over. The categorization of clients is based on the nature of their most recent ES contact only (so combination cases are eliminated). Detailed analysis of the social, economic, and health situation of these sub-groups follows, based on our coding of both client history data and data from the client assessments.

Compared to the random sample of housing risk clients, the interviewed sub-sample contains significantly more blacks, more people living in their own homes or apartments at last ES contact, and more with multiple referrals to ES and with more recorded problems. (Those in their own residences on whom more information was available were easier to locate.) The number of problems and number of ES referrals are the same for the located and non-located groups, although the located clients are also somewhat younger and are less likely to have been undomiciled at the last ES contact. The located clients looked much like those who were not located on gender, age, marital status, proportion undomiciled at last ES contact, and proportion living in SROs, and thus we can be fairly confident in generalizing to the housing risk from the interviews on certain dimensions.

Comparing the Shelter, Housing Conditions and the SRO interviewees we find the SRO sub-group has more males, is younger, and is less likely to be married or widowed. They are also receiving substantially more informal help, are more mentally intact, and have relatively low levels of need (as indicated by relatively low scores on the OARS assessment instrument). Thus, as was expected, the SRO clients are substantially better off than are the ES clients.

Placement in Shelters

Having "need for shelter" as a problem did not necessarily mean that clients had been placed in shelter, and clients who had other needs sometimes were placed in shelter. Investigation revealed that 83% of those clients identified as needing shelter actually had used it. However, 25% of those with poor housing conditions also had used shelter. Clients who use shelter, however, were found to have significantly more problems cited in the case record ($p = .006$) and more referrals to ES ($p = .0001$).

"Shelter" was defined as any agency provided housing which by its own definition is temporary, including both overnight and transitional shelters which have limits on the duration of stay. Our definition also includes hotels and other facilities (e.g., rooming houses, congregate living facilities and nursing homes) where clients are placed by city agencies for shelter, as well as transitional shelters that have the potential of becoming permanent situations. Most of the "senior shelters" utilized by ES do, in fact, allow and even facilitate their shelter clients in becoming permanent residents. This raises a complicated question about when shelter becomes no longer temporary, but has effectively become a home. For empirical purposes, we determined that as long as DHS was still paying for the shelter stay it was using emergency shelter funds, and so we would consider the placement temporary. (The difficulty is in the normative issue of saying at what point shelter, in fact, becomes a permanent placement and when should DHS stop paying for it. As will be shown, shelter is a resolution utilized inordinately often for certain clients because so few other options are available.)

A substantial proportion of those "needing shelter" present no evidence that they ever used or were placed in a public shelter.

Reasons that these clients had not used shelter fall into two general categories – client initiated and system or agency initiated. Examples of client initiated reasons for not using shelter are that the client refused it or that the client disappeared before receiving services. Examples of system initiated reasons include the shelters being full, shelters refusing to admit certain clients for some other reason, and clients' homes being located. For housing condition clients, reasons for non-use are more likely to be system initiated, mainly that if any alternative residence existed ES was less likely to place the client in city paid shelter. For clients in need of shelter, reasons are more likely to be client initiated, including refusals and disappearances.

Forty-five percent of the individuals who used shelter were not really "homeless" except by definition of being in a shelter. In other words, there appeared to be other housing in which they were living, but it was uninhabitable, unenterable, too unsafe or unhealthy, or could not be located. This finding requires a closer look at the connection between homelessness and the use of shelter for these persons. We find some non-congruence between use of shelter and "homelessness" which is discussed later.

Homelessness

The study examines three dimensions of homelessness: whether the individual was ever homeless and is still homeless; whether homelessness is short-term or long-term; and whether it is a single episode or is repeated. We were interested in the extent to which all three of the housing risk groups have experienced homelessness, whether they are currently or had ever been homeless and the duration of that homelessness.

Homelessness was distinguished by its duration, with "current" being at the time of the researchers' contact and interview, "ever" meaning ever in the respondent's adult life, and "never" being just that. Using the definition operationalized by Sosin and associates (p. 22), with some additional parameters (in brackets), we defined "homelessness" as: (1) residing for up to two weeks with a friend or relative, not paying rent, and not being sure that the stay would surpass fourteen days; (2) residing in a shelter [or other agency-paid temporary housing]; (3) being without normal, acceptable shelter arrangements and thus sleeping out-of-doors; or (4) residing in a treatment center for the indigent for less than ninety days [e.g., a hospital, detox, mental health, halfway house, or shelter for battered women] and claiming to have no place to go. To further refine this, in keeping with Kutza's criterion, "long-term homelessness" is defined as being homeless continuously or repeatedly for a period of one year or longer.

Of the 94 ES clients and 27 SRO clients for whom data are available, 50% of the ES clients and 80% of the SRO clients were found to have never been homeless. Of all those interviewed, 51% were homeless at one time. Of these, a third were homeless more than once and 28% had experienced long-term homelessness. Of all those who had experienced homelessness, over half were homeless only once and only briefly.

Being homeless, however, does not mean that the older person had stayed in a shelter. Of the 55 interviewed individuals who had been homeless at some time, 49% had actually stayed at a shelter. Of those who did not use shelter, nearly two-thirds avoided placement themselves, usually because family or friends too them in or they found other arrangements. For one-fifth it distinctly appeared that the service system had not provided the shelter they may have needed. For one-seventh, both client and system initiated reasons operated to prevent the use of shelter. This begins to indicate the severe constraints and discretion under which provisions are made even for those already identified to be at substantial risk.

Comparisons of the ever- and never-homeless groups reveal no statistically significant demographic differences. In terms of frequency of homelessness, however, having been homeless once, blacks are significantly more likely to have additional periods of homelessness ($t = 2.01$, $df = 46$, $p = .050$).

Two other problems that correlate significantly with homelessness are a history of evictions and evidence of impaired mental functioning. The latter problem includes dementia, but also mental illness and depression which are readily misperceived as dementia. Alcohol or drug abuse, while present among over three-quarters of those who were ever homeless, is not significantly more common among them. Being burned out, handicapped, or abused also show no significant differences in frequency between the ever- and never-homeless.

Resources Make a Difference

Social factors normally considered to be of support to older persons were also examined, including the number of children, contact with children, living with others, and availability of formal or informal helpers. These specific factors show no significant differences between the homeless and the never homeless groups when considered one at a time. However, significant differences are found in some of the dimensions of the OARS evaluation that was used to assess the resources and functional level of the interviewed sample.

Individuals who were never homeless scored significantly better in total social resources, mental health status, activities of daily living, and in the composite total OARS score than those who were currently or had been homeless. The never homeless also have significantly larger incomes, a mean average of $595 as opposed to $434. They also present evidence of significantly less dementia (see Table 3.4) as scored on the Portable Mental Status Questionnaire. We found no significant differences in physical health, or in specific economic resources other than monthly income. It appears, then, that it is largely certain critical *combinations* of deficits in resources, as well as in environmental circumstances, that determine who among the elderly is insulated from homelessness. Critical factors that have been identified here are of an endogenous nature only and include deficits in cognitive and mental capacity, monthly income, and the availability of social support or assistance.

When the SRO group is compared with the ES group, on average they show better overall functioning. Regardless of whether or not they were ever homeless, the SRO group is less likely to have had children, or to be in touch with their children; more are helped by neighbors or hotel staff rather than by relatives; and on average they have higher monthly incomes than ES clients. Although they are younger than the ES clients, their "better off" status is not explained by this either. They appear to be supported by some nontraditional factors which are explored further in Chapter 8.

In conclusion then, the interview data suggests that the higher incidence of dementia and lower monthly incomes and lack of social support, sharply distinguish the ever homeless and the never homeless. The compounding effects of the lack of resources of all types, as indicated by the total OARS score, are also important. The

Table 3.4. Resources by Whether or Not Ever Homeless

Variable	Group	n	Value	df	t	p
mean income	Never Ever	37 38	595 434	56	2.23	.030*
Social resources score	Never Ever	37 39	2.62 3.54	74	-3.14	.002*
Economic Resource score	Never Ever	36 38	3.03 3.33	72	-1.2.	.235
Mental health score	Never Ever	37 40	2.68 3.30	75	-2.70	.009*
Physical Health score	Never Ever	37 38	3.49 3.59	73	-0.51	.610
ADL score	Never Ever	37 39	2.76 3.32	74	-2.02	.047*
Total OARS score	Never Ever	35 36	14.3 17.1	69	-3.73	.000*
Mean dementia score	Never Ever	36 36	1.31 1.92	56	-2.94	.005*

SRO residents as a group, while having equally poor health and economic resources, appear to be better off generally because of the social support and contact available in their immediate surroundings.

Finally, the stability of client residential history and outcome was examined to assess the stability of interviewees' current living arrangement and trace the stability of past living arrangements. As can be seen on Tables 3.5 and 3.6, the living arrangements of the never-homeless were significantly more stable at the time of the research interview ($p = .04$), and had been more stable in the past ($p = .0001$), than persons who had ever been homeless. Those who had been homeless exhibited a significantly higher level of housing instability with patterns of evictions, relocations and returns to shelters and the streets.

Finally, we were eager to confirm where the 126 ES clients had "ended up" at last known contact but can only report on the 91 who were actually located. At least 20% of the total ES sample were confirmed to have died and another 20% were incapable of contributing significantly to the interview.

Of the 19 who had been undomiciled at the time of the last ES contact, 7 were still undomiciled when our researchers contacted them. Of the other undomiciled clients, the last known living arrangements were found to be:

Hospital	3
Nursing home	3
Board and Care	1
Congregate housing	1
Own apartment	2
Unknown	2

Comparing histories of homelessness on only those (approximately 75) for whom it could be confirmed, eight (18%) of the ever-homeless had died as had 9 (20%) of the never homeless.

Table 3.5. Stability of Last Living Arrangement

	Never	Ever
Stable	41	27
Change immanent	3	9
Change forseeable	8	12
Not applicable		1
Not known	3	8

Chi^2=9.92, df=4, p=.04

Table 3.6. Stability of Living Arrangements Over Time

	Never	Ever
Past and current	36	11
Current only	3	8
Past only	6	19
Chronic instability		8
Not clear, unknown	10	11

chi^2=30, df=4, p=.0000

Thus, of that small group of clients who had had repeated contact with ES and who could be found, at least one in three are still on the streets after one to four years. Less than a third are in room and board facilities or independent housing. The rest had died or become institutionalized. Very few ever really resettled. This suggests that this very small but troubling group, the elderly chronically undomiciled, is very difficult to move into normal and permanent housing.

SUMMARY

Statistical analysis of the demographic characteristics of the random sample indicate that black elderly, the poor, and individuals over 75 years of age are over-represented among elderly emergency clients. Emergencies among the elderly appear to occur unevenly across the city. Neighborhoods having an abundance of run down housing show the most seniors in deplorable conditions, and neighborhoods with a shortage of low rent housing show the most need for temporary housing and emergency shelter (not to mention affordable permanent housing). About half of elderly ES clients present only one problem, and nearly four-fifths are seen by ES only once. Most commonly occurring problems are fires, being lost of confused, needing transportation, and needing temporary shelter. Housing related incidents account for at least 47% of all elderly emergencies that merit city attention, and probably closer to 75%. Only 7% of the clients are referred to ES four or more times, suggesting that the vast majority cope in emergencies largely on their own, and that a very small and very needy population having serious resource deficits make substantial demands on city emergency programs.

Multi-referral clients have multiple problems including, for at least a third of them, a need for temporary shelter. Housing related problems are very persistent, with shelter need persisting from the first to the last contact in 68% of the cases and poor housing conditions persisting for 33%.

Data on services reveal that shelter is provided by ES to seniors for a wide variety of problems. Most shelter use is of limited duration but a small group of elderly shelter users stay or repeatedly reenter shelters for a period longer than one year. When elders need shelter but are not placed, reasons have as much to do with agency inability (and sometimes unwillingness) to place them as with client unwillingness to leave a deplorable home.

Client assessments of those who were interviewed reveal that ES clients with housing related problems are substantially worse off than SRO residents despite having similar levels of economic resources and health problems. A major difference between them is the higher level of cognitive impairment found among the ES clients.

ES clients have more than twice the incidence of episodes of actual homelessness as do SRO clients. Of both groups, thirty-three percent of the clients who have ever been homeless are homeless more than once, and 28% experience long-term homelessness. Problems that correlate with homelessness are a history of evictions, current cognitive impairment (usually dementia), severely limited monthly income, and lack of available social resources.

Finally, analysis of the ES clients' recent living arrangements indicate that at least 20% of them have died and a similar number have been institutionalized in the one to four years following their most recent ES contact. While this may not be an excessive proportion given their ages, the gravity of their circumstances is revealed in the extent to which many of those who died appear to have suffered substantial and preventable trauma and medical conditions. Elders who have required emergency interventions from the city are a population that is very difficult to ever move back into normal, decent housing.

In Chapter 5 we discuss some of the tragic events that led to many of these deaths. Keeping these descriptive parameters in mind we examine the unique patterns in the experience of older individuals who have been assisted by Emergency Services. We are extremely grateful to the individuals who have provided this information, but have attempted to preserve their privacy. With the exception of identified agencies and one of the hotels, all names have been altered in the following chapters.

Before describing the individuals located in the study just described, the next chapter will examine in detail a population of "traditional homeless" elderly persons who were investigated in Detroit through a quite different method than the one just described. Rather than use agency records and then track down the clients, that study used a field survey of places frequented by homeless persons. The study addresses that relatively small group of chronically undomiciled elderly, mainly men, who were least likely to be found in the Chicago study. The larger sample in Detroit supplements the present description with several important characteristics and problems of chronically homeless older men.

REFERENCES

Kutza, E. (1987). *Undomiciled elderly persons in Chicago*. Park Ridge: Retirement Research Foundation.

Sosin, M., Colson, P. & Grossman, S. (1988). *Homelessness in Chicago*. Chicago: School of Social Service Administration, The University of Chicago and Chicago Community Trust.

Chapter 4

Racial Differences Regarding Shelter and Housing in a Sample of Urban Elderly Homeless

Richard L. Douglass
Benjamin J. Hodgkins

SUMMARY. A sample of elderly homeless persons in Detroit is discussed with an emphasis on distinctions between black and white racial strata. The analyses, based on a field survey conducted in 1988, reveal that several variables distinguish racial groups, including social relationships and kinship, frequency and duration of homelessness, and previous institutional experiences. Economic differences were not found between black and white elderly homeless persons. White homeless elderly resemble the traditional homeless men who are the subjects of many urban sociological studies of skid row, while the black elderly homeless are presented as a newly emerged subset of homelessness.

INTRODUCTION

Complex issues associated with homelessness, both as a social issue and as a personal tragedy, have confronted the United States in recent years. Homelessness is a stark reminder that economic growth without social and economic distributive justice will leave behind people with various social, physical or emotional disabilities

---

Richard L. Douglass, MPH, PhD, is affiliated with the College of Health and Human Services, Eastern Michigan University, Ypsilanti, MI 48197.

Benjamin J. Hodgkins, PhD, is affiliated with the School of Medicine, Wayne State University, Detroit, MI 48201.

The authors wish to thank the Detroit Area Agency on Aging and the Michigan Office of Services to the Aging for supporting the research reported here.

who have inadequate or absent supportive resources upon which to depend. Efforts to provide assistance to these groups frequently assume that they are homogeneous in their needs, although considerable evidence exists to suggest that such is not the case. Thus, most recent inquiries about the homeless focus on what is generally referred to as the "new homeless"; families set adrift by the closure of factories or displaced by other sources of job loss and reductions in the availability of affordable housing (Kroll et al., 1986, Rossi et al., 1986; Bassuk, Rubin and Lauriat, 1986). Also, as graphically described by Kozol (1988), the new urban homeless are largely young adults whose personal problems with drugs, alcohol, chronic poverty, family violence or criminal behavior have excluded them from mainstream community life.

The more traditional homeless have been largely males with chronic alcohol abuse, histories of criminal behavior, lack of familial supports, and mental health problems (Andersen, 1923; Dunham, 1953; Bogue, 1963; Levinson, 1963; Bahr and Lanfur, 1967; Cohen and Sokolovsky, 1983. The traditional homeless have been called Skid Row bums, derelicts or other derogatory names and have been the subject of a significant sociological and anthropological literature (Wallace, 1965). The traditional homeless, as described in these studies, rarely includes women; the image is virtually always a male who is "down and out." The traditional homeless, however, have not been the subjects of major national attention, as have been the new homeless of the last decade; social services and legislative solutions have never been as substantial for the traditional homeless as informal and private charitable services. While the elderly may comprise a relatively small proportion of the new homeless, they are far more significant among the traditionally homeless. The social and emotional needs of both groups differ, yet programs available to them tend not to be designed to distinguish such differences.

The following discussion will summarize the methods and principle findings of a field study of homeless elderly people in Detroit (Douglass et al., 1988), as they relate to the programmatic needs of the elderly, which are quite different from the "new homeless" or the young adult. To further explore the heterogeneity of this elderly homeless sample, these data will be analyzed in terms of racial differences. The analyses and their implications will be discussed in consideration of the need for greater sensitivity to the diverse backgrounds of the homeless in order to plan and provide meaningful services, outreach programs and to develop prevention strategies for the growing problem of homelessness in American society.

REPORT SUMMARY AND ANALYSES BY RACE

No group of individuals present a more compelling image of personal hardship than the elderly homeless who exist in urban centers throughout the country. Although most investigators have found that the elderly constitute a relatively small proportion of the total homeless population, for the oldest among them this is likely to be a chronic condition; a population of people who have often been unable to acquire or sustain a permanent home or reliable shelter for many years. At least in this respect they tend to differ from the majority of today's homeless. From our work in Detroit we have concluded that a large proportion of these elderly homeless persons (who we operationally define as at least 55 years old) have been without traditional, stable housing for a large portion of their adult lives.

To the extent that the elderly homeless are characteristically chronic in their condition of homelessness, they fit much of the stereotype associated with the history of becoming homeless. From the limited available research, which has been largely descriptive in nature, a common picture of the psychosocial factors related to homelessness and the homeless has emerged. Social factors, such as abject poverty, associated with the loss of low income housing due to urban decay and/or gentrification of urban neighborhoods, are related to unemployment or precipitous job loss, little formal education, limited employment potential, and personal histories of tragedy and failure. These conditions in turn are frequently accentuated by an individual's history of mental illness, drug or alcohol addiction, criminal behavior and/or criminal victimization. These observations are consistent with those of others, including Wright and Weber (1987) and Gelberg, Linn and Leake (1988).

Research Design and Generalizability

At the request of the Michigan Office of Services to the Aging, the Detroit Area Agency on Aging commissioned a study of Detroit's elderly homeless population in 1988. The six month study was conducted between April and September of that year. The design included a primary sample of 56 locations in Detroit where homeless persons were known to congregate, according to a panel of aging services providers. From this list of 56 locations initial site visits indicated that only 19 sites were frequented by homeless persons who were at least 55 years old on a regular basis. At each of these 19 primary sample sites potential respondents were screened according to age, and housing status; of approximately 900 persons who were screened 119 interviews were completed. Of these, 85 interviews were found to be complete, appropriate and suitable for statistical analysis. Absence of a place to live, dependence on temporary shelter arrangements, and self-professed homelessness were the principal inclusion criteria, in addition to age being over 55. Data collection was accomplished by personal interviews, using a pretested survey instrument and trained interviewers. The instrument was a composite of questions previously used in aging services needs assessment surveys in Michigan and field studies of the homeless in other cities. It is fully described in the study's final technical report (Douglass et al., 1988).

The resulting purposive sample represents a population of homeless elderly persons who make use of shelter, clothing, food, or other services and the parks and other places in Detroit where homeless elderly persons congregate during the summer months. It does not represent those persons who never frequent the places where data were collected, such as people who find shelter in basements of abandoned buildings and do not seek companionship or services in the primary sample sites that were used. In this study, due to limited resources and security of the field staff, no attempt was made to explore all vacant buildings, alleys, vacant lots and other places where homeless persons might be found. For purposes of generalizability, this sample is best described as a sample of places, with representative interviews at each location. It is not appropriate to use this sample to extrapolate the prevalence of homelessness among Detroit's elderly or to assume that this sample is completely representative of the city's elderly homeless.

FINDINGS: DIFFERENCES BETWEEN BLACK AND WHITE RESPONDENTS

The 85 complete interviews included 17 women and 68 men. Of the women, nine were white and eight were black. Twenty-five of the men were white, 40 were black and 3 were hispanic. This is an over-representation of black persons in the sample in that less than 50% of Detroit's population over age 60 is black, versus 55% of this sample.

The age distribution of the sample ranged from 54 to 86, with a mean age of 62.1 and standard deviation of 6.6. Thus, this sample of elderly homeless persons is largely composed of the "young old." While the reasons for this have not been investigated thoroughly, it is at least reasonable to speculate that with increasing age the effects of mortality, institutional placement, or benefits of income entitlements contribute to pathways out of the homeless condition. In the Detroit sample there was a dramatic decrease in the numbers of elderly homeless persons above age 65.

The economic status of this sample can be most simply described as a metaphor for all other findings about these people, with 42.7% stating that they had less than $200 for all of their needs during the preceding month. The maximum income was slightly over $600 (including only seven individuals). The sample was seriously impoverished, rarely participated in any form or pension, entitlement, or income maintenance program. The most usual source of income (44%) was collecting bottles and cans for recovery of the cash deposit of $.10 (in Michigan). No statistically significant differences were measured when the average monthly income was assessed according to the respondent's race. For both black and white respondents, approximately 75% reported monthly income of under $400.

From this sample, it became clear that the elderly homeless of Detroit, like homeless people of other age groups and in other places, are largely unattached individuals. The largest group of the sample were either never married, divorced, or separated, accounting for 68.6% of the respondents. Nineteen percent were widowed and 7% (all men) claimed that they were married, although there was no evidence that their spouse was available for an interview. Four men reported that they had been abandoned by their wives. Respondents who reported the lowest monthly incomes, moreover, were also most likely to be single and never married, separated, divorced or abandoned.

When considered according to race, different marital patterns appear between white and black respondents. While comparable proportions of the white and black samples reported being married, divorced, separated or abandoned, black respondents were three times as likely to be widowed as white respondents, while white respondents were twice as likely as their black counterparts to be single and never married.

Residency and Homelessness

All except three of the respondents in this study claimed to be residents of Detroit and 85% indicated that they had lived in the city for more than five years. Only eight respondents (9.4%) suggested that they would stay in Detroit for six months or less, while over 72% indicated that they planned to stay for more than a year. Respondents were directly asked if they had a place which was a permanent home and how long it had been since they lived there. While 53% of the respondents claimed to have a regular place to call home, none of them planned to sleep in that place on the night of the interview. The importance of "having a place" was clear to these people, even if the meaning was far from conventional. No differences were found in these measures between black and white respondents.

Among the respondents, on the night of the interview, 23% planned to sleep in a hotel room, 24% were staying in a shelter or a rescue mission, 24% expected to sleep in a friend's or relative's home and 30% either did not know where they would sleep or planned to sleep in some other place such as a park, hotel lobby, under a bridge, in an abandoned car, or in a vacant building. These data were collected during a very hot and dry summer and it can be presumed that in less hospitable weather the options for shelter would have been somewhat different.

The most recent source of temporary shelter also revealed differences between white and black respondents. Table 1 compares black and white use of hotel/SRO, a formal shelter program, the residence of a friend or an aggregated "other" category that represented a wide range of non-conventional places, such as space under bridges, bus or train stations, parks, abandoned buildings and other public places. In this table the differences in white and black use of hotel/SRO and the various "other" sources of shelter are minimal, however, white respondents were more likely to use the residence of a friend than a formal shelter program, while black respondents were more likely to utilize a shelter.

Having a "place to stay" and having a home is not the same thing for these respondents. Still, among the 46 percent that claimed to have a regular place to call home, 13% had been there within one week and 13% had not been there in one year or longer. Individuals who did not have a place that they considered to be their home were likely to have been without a home for more than a

TABLE 1. RESPONDENT'S MOST RECENT SOURCE OF TEMPORARY SHELTER, BY RACE (within-race percentages)

	White		Black	
	n	%	n	%
Hotel/SRO	7	21.9	11	23.4
Shelter	6	18.8	12	25.5
Friend	9	28.1	10	21.3
Other *	10	31.3	14	29.8
	n = 32		n = 47	

* Public place, abandoned building, park, under a bridge, abandoned car or bus

month and over 40% of them had been homeless for a year or longer. Fifty-four percent of the respondents either stated that they did not have specific plans for a place to stay in the near future or simply didn't know if such a prospect was possible. When the respondent's race was considered in association with these questions regarding the availability of a home, or "regular" place to stay, no statistically significant differences were found. In the sample 51.5% of the black respondents and 55.3% of the white respondents were without such a place to call their own. Given the difficulty respondents had acknowledging this condition, we consider these proportions to be conservative.

The prevailing condition among these people was a long period of homelessness and an uncertain likelihood of known housing in the future. In addition, more than half of the respondents indicated that their last regular home was one in which they lived alone, rather than with someone else and, of these individuals, 59% had not lived with anyone else for five or more years. When considered according to race, in their last regular home 60.6% of the white respondents lived with someone else compared to only 40.4% of the black respondents.

The frequency and duration of homelessness was different between black and white elderly respondents. Approximately one third of the sample had been homeless in each of the four years prior to the interview (1984-1987) and a quarter of the respondents had been homeless for up to twenty years. While about 44% of the white respondents stated that this was their first experience with homelessness, almost 64% of the black respondents said that this was their initial homeless experience. Sixty percent of the black respondents reported that the time of the interview was their first experience with homelessness, while almost 55% of the white respondents reported multiple homeless experiences.

The duration of homelessness reflects this racial contrast, as well as shown in Table 2. Respondents were asked, "Is this the first time you have been without a regular place to live?" and [If "no"] "Were you without a regular place to live in: 1987, 1986, 1985, 1984, other times?" The proportion of white respondents who were homeless in 1987, 1986 and 1985 in addition to the 1988 date of the interview was 94%, while 76% of these individuals were homeless

TABLE 2. RESPONDENTS FOR WHOM 1988 WAS NOT THEIR INITIAL HOMELESSNESS - Recent experiences without a regular place to live, by race and year (within-race percentages of respondents for whom current situation was not their first experience with homelessness)

	White n=17 (51% of White Total Sample)		Black n=15 (31% of Black Total Sample)	
1987	16	(94%)	14	(93%)
1986	16		12	(80%)
1985	16		11	(73%)
1984	13	(76%)	11	
Before 1984	13		6	(40%)

in 1984 and prior to that. By the same measures 93% of the black respondents who were homeless in 1988 were also homeless in 1987. This percentage decreased, however, in each of the previous time periods for these respondents, with 12% homeless in 1986, 11% in 1985 and 1984, and only 6% before 1984.

Social Relationships and Support

In general, these long-term homeless respondents had little contact with a nuclear family situation in recent years. The respondents who had last lived with someone else were most likely (30%) to have lived with a spouse. The homes of other relatives (21%), friends (18%) and unrelated adults (10%) were the other sources of temporary housing for this subset of the sample. Only 8% of these elderly poor had ever lived with their children. Seven individuals had not lived with anyone else since they left their original nuclear family as youths, suggesting that a solitary life style at a young age can, for some, portend solitude in advanced age.

One of the dynamics of homelessness, as suggested earlier in this discussion, is the relationship of the homeless elderly to other people. It is already clear that these people do not have an abundance of social supports and kinship, but does this generality apply equally to black and white elderly homeless? Table 3 presents data that indicate that 64.5% of the white respondents had lived with someone else, compared to only 43.2% of the black respondents. And of those who had lived with someone else, virtually identical proportions of black and white respondents had previously lived with a spouse or an unrelated adult. However, black respondents were more likely to have been living with their own children or with other relatives (35% compared to 24.1% for white respondents) while white respondents were more likely to have lived with friends (20.7% compared to 12.5% for black respondents). Thus there appears to have been a qualitative as well as a quantitative difference between black and white respondents; white elderly homeless persons were more likely than black to have lived with someone else and most often that was a friend. Black respondents, less likely to have lived with someone else, were more likely than white respondents to have lived with relatives.

The apparent difference between black and white respondents regarding proximity of residence with relatives versus friends or unrelated adults was further explored, however the sample contained

TABLE 3. PERCENTAGE OF RESPONDENTS WHO, IN THEIR LAST PERMANENT HOME, LIVED ALONE OR WITH SOMEONE ELSE, BY RACE (within-race percentages)

	White		Black	
	n	%	n	%
Lived alone	11	35.5	25	56.8
Lived with someone else	20	64.5	19	43.2
	n = 31		n = 44	

very few white respondents who claimed to have relatives living in the Detroit Metropolitan area. Given the small numbers, the analyses are presented in Tables 4 and 5. The data in Table 4 show that of the 9 white respondents who verified that they did have relatives living in the Detroit area, only 2 stated that they would "be in favor of going to live with them," while 7 of the 18 black respondents with geographically proximal relatives would be in favor of going

TABLE 4. WOULD RESPONDENT BE OPPOSED TO OR IN FAVOR OF MOVING INTO THE HOME OF RELATIVES LIVING IN THE DETROIT AREA? BY RACE, FOR THOSE WITH RELATIVES LIVING WITHIN THE DETROIT METROPOLITAN AREA (within-race percentages)

	White n=9	Black n=18
Opposed	44.4%	50.0%
In favor	22.2%	38.9%
Don't know or refused	22.2%	5.6%

TABLE 5. WOULD THE RESPONDENT'S RELATIVES BE OPPOSED TO OR IN FAVOR OF HAVING THE RESPONDENT MOVE INTO THEIR HOME? BY RACE, for those respondents with relatives within the metropolitan Detroit area (within-race percentages)

	White n=9	Black n=18
Opposed	44.4%	27.8%
In Favor	33.3%	61.1%
Don't Know or Refused	11.1%	11.1%

to live with them. Similarly, in Table 5, when asked if their relatives would be receptive to the respondent "moving in with them" 44.4% of the white respondents, compared to 27.8% of the black respondents, indicated that their relatives would be opposed to such a proposition. It appears reasonable to speculate that within the considerable isolation of the homeless elderly in Detroit, the black respondents were, as a group, not as thoroughly estranged from familial ties as the white respondents. This question would require a larger sample to properly explore.

SUMMARY OF FINDINGS

The institutional experience of this sample, when examined by race, revealed clear distinctions in places where the respondents had been at a significant or total loss of personal control and hints at differences in both behavioral characteristics of the sample and, to an extent, how society has dealt with these individuals in their earlier lives. Racial differences in alcohol or drug detoxification, mental hospital admission, State or Federal prison time and local jail detention were highly significant as shown in Table 6. Black respondents were more likely to have been in drug or alcohol detoxification (principally alcohol), far less likely to have been admitted to a mental hospital, and more likely to have served time in a State or

TABLE 6. RESPONDENT INSTITUTIONAL EXPERIENCES BY RACE (within-race percentages)

	White		Black	
	n	%	n	%
Alcohol or Drug Detoxification (inpatient)	7	21	16	34
Mental Hospital Admission	17	52	9	19
State or Federal Prison Time	4	12	14	30
City or County Jail Time	11	33	26	55

Federal prison or a local jail than white respondents. Over half of the white sample had been admitted to a mental hospital (52%) while only 19% of the black respondents verified such an experience.

DISCUSSION

All available research on the elderly homeless is substantially parochial, being conducted usually in only one city. The present study of the Detroit elderly homeless is no exception. Accordingly, the extent to which these research findings are appropriately generalized to other places is limited. In our opinion places cannot be assumed to be comparable because of political, economic and local historical factors that affect the nature and extent of poverty, tolerance to the presence of homeless people and the extent of social response to them. Thus, this research on this subject should be considered as suggestive, but clearly not definitive, regarding the characteristics of the homeless elderly.

Much of the literature of the homeless in America is noted for ironies that emerge from the detailed analysis of racial distinctions. In Detroit, while only about 35% of the population over age 70 is black, the majority of the homeless elderly are black. Unlike the larger community, among the poorest of the poor who are homeless, there appears to be little difference between black and white. Nonetheless, there are distinctions revealed in the present analyses that may assist thoughtful planners and service providers to develop methods of preventing homelessness or finding housing alternatives for the most vulnerable elderly.

The white elderly homeless in this sample were most likely to have been single and never married and to have been homeless for many years. Black elderly homeless respondents were twice as likely as white respondents to have been widowed and to have been homeless for less than four years. White respondents were more likely to have most recently lived with someone else who was most often a friend. By contrast the black elderly homeless most recently lived alone, but their most recent living arrangement with anyone else was either a relative or one of their adult children.

From very limited information it may be true that black elderly homeless respondents were more likely than white respondents to regard living with a geographically available relative acceptable and, if sought, would result in acceptance by relatives. Very few white respondents, however, acknowledged the availability of any relatives in the metropolitan Detroit area. If it is true that the black elderly homeless have a higher probability of residual ties to relatives, then seeking temporary shelter or a more permanent alternative may be a more productive option for them, on the average, than with their elderly white counterparts.

Probably the most striking distinction between black and white respondents in this study is their prior experience in institutions. Black respondents were far more likely than white respondents to have served time in jail and prison, while white respondents were more frequently former patients in state mental hospitals. While the causal relationship, if any, between a personal history in one of these "total institutions" and the homeless condition has yet to be proven independent of other contributing factors, the strength of the distinction is not likely to be dismissed by the introduction of other variables. We believe there may be productive use of this information to more thoroughly understand the causes of homelessness and to develop programs to preclude homelessness among the elderly in the future. Thus, former mental patients may have different linkages to governmental and community resources than former prisoners, while prisoners' linkages to kinship and family systems may be different than those of former mental hospital patients. If so, perhaps such differences could be addressed in a way that would give more opportunity for each group to adjust to community life upon release from the institution.

In this analysis, we have sought to demonstrate that elderly homeless are not homogeneous. In spite of many apparent similarities, social and historical conditions can contribute to a diversity of needs within groups such as the elderly homeless. Thus, white elderly respondents in this study are reminiscent of the traditional homeless of the urban anthropological studies of isolated men, skid row and related subjects. Black elderly respondents, on the other hand, tend to reflect both a different pattern of previous experience in society and more enduring social relationships. The implications of these differences for possible alleviation of homelessness among the elderly should not be ignored.

Urban renewal, residential flight to suburban communities and other frequently noted dynamics of urban centers will likely continue. As urban centers decay and are transformed into places which are alien to the elderly poor, this pattern should become more commonplace among the elderly homeless. Such a prospect should, at the least, stimulate new and more thorough investigations which will lead to programs which take advantage of information gleaned from such efforts. Then it may be possible to plan more effective responses to the variety of human needs found among the homeless population.

REFERENCES

Andersen, N. The Hobo: The Sociology of the Homeless Man. Chicago: The University of Chicago Press, 1923.

Bogue, D. Skid Row in American Cities. Chicago: The University of Chicago, 1963.

Bussuk, E.L., L. Rubin and A. Lauriat. "Characteristics of Sheltered Homeless Families." American Journal of Public Health. 76: 1097-1101, 1986.

Cohen, C.I. and J. Sokolovsky. "Toward a Concept of Homelessness Among Aged Men." Journal of Gerontology. 38: 81-89, 1983.

Douglass, R.L., B.J. Atchison, W.J. Lofton and B.J. Hodgkins. Aged, Adrift and Alone: Detroit's Elderly Homeless. Ypsilanti, MI: Eastern Michigan University, 1988.

Dunham, W.H. Homeless Men and Their Habitats. Detroit: Wayne State University, 1953.

Gelberg, L., L.S. Linn, and B.D. Leake. "Mental Health, Alcohol and Drug Use, and Criminal History Among Homeless Adults." American Journal of Psychiatry. 145: 191-196, 1988.

Kozol, J. Rachel and Her Children: Homeless Families in America. New York: Crown Publishers, Inc. 1988.

Kroll, J., K. Carvey, D. Hagadorn, P. Firedog, and E. Banavides. "A Survey of Homeless Adults in Urban Emergency Shelters." Hospital and Community Psychiatry. 37: 283-286, 1986.

Levinson, B. "The Homeless Man: A Psychological Enigma." Mental Hygiene. 47: 590-602, 1963.

Rossi, P.H., G.A. Fisher and G. Willis. The Condition of the Homeless of Chicago. Amherst: Social and Demographic Research Institute, 1986.

Wallace, S.E. Skid Row as a Way of Life. Totowa: The Bedminster Press, Inc., 1965.

Wright, J.D. and E. Weber. Homelessness and Health. Washington, D.C.: McGraw-Hill, Inc., 1987.

Chapter 5

The Emergency Service Clients: Coping with Threats to and Loss of "Home"

Rebecca Hanson Berman
Sharon M. Keigher

SUMMARY. Several housing risk clients identified in Chapter 3 are profiled here in detail regarding their housing circumstances and how they have been coping with these problems. Individuals are described for whom dislocation was brief; for whom homelessness was long term, repeated or habitual; or who have never been without a home. Most persons in the latter category are subsisting in this state at substantial personal risk. The unique coping abilities of each type are highlighted.

Leo Tolstoy began his novel *Anna Karenina* with the observation, "Happy families are all alike; every unhappy family is unhappy in its own way." And so it is with elderly persons faced with imminent loss of their homes or their independence: the variations in their individual circumstances and coping capacities are unlimited.

Interpretation of statistical analyses alone cannot convey the overwhelming significance, pathos, and complexity of these individuals' circumstances, nor their strengths and fierce survival instincts of the seniors identified in the previous chapters. To do so more meaningfully, this chapter presents several profiles of the elderly ES clients who were described in Chapter 3, including general descriptions of the commonalities and variations in their housing problem situations from a more holistic, in-context perspective.

These cases highlight several issues and emerging themes in the lives of older individuals who have experienced serious, sometimes life threatening housing related emergencies. Examination of how individuals cope in the face of housing difficulties offers valuable information on how it is that some become homeless and some do not. This qualitative description suggests the meaning that housed and homeless situations have for elderly people.

These cases and general descriptions are organized around elderly persons who have ever been homeless and those who have never been homeless. Within each category brief attention is given to different kinds of homelessness, different kinds of housing situations and different patterns of relocations. Preliminary analysis of their coping abilities suggests wide variation in the receptivity of the elderly to service interventions and in their reasons for use of shelters.

COPING ABILITIES OF THE HOMELESS

The One Time, Short Term Homeless

Contrary to much that has been written about the homeless elderly, our sample does not focus on the "chronic traditional homeless" (Doolin, 1986) or the long term skid row population (Cohen & Sokolovsky, 1989; Douglass, 1988). The majority of the cases of homelessness reported in Chapter 3 are individuals who were homeless only once for relatively short periods of time. Many of the one time homeless drew on formal and informal social resources to pull themselves out of their homeless state and, as was indicated earlier, most are no longer homeless. The sometimes multiple events surrounding slippage into homelessness include evictions, fires, loss of social supports, loss of income (e.g., due to a robbery or loss of a spouse's income), inability to manage funds due to diminished mental capacities or alcoholism, fears or paranoia resulting in a self-initiated move, and so on. In addition, the ability of individuals to cope in both preventing and finding a route out of homelessness varies considerably.

The following case description illustrates the inability of an elderly woman to cope in the face of diminishing social (and probably economic) resources and encroaching dementia. These resulted in the loss of her home, her subsequent adaptation to shelter life and efforts to maintain a sense of "home."

Josie Hicks: Homeless in Her Own Home

Josie Hicks, 85 years old, presents a case of ill-defined homelessness in some ways complicated by those attempting to help her. From Josie's perspective, she was never homeless and still has her home. She is homeless by our definitions because legally she no longer owns her home and because she was placed against her will in a shelter where she still resides. We found Josie, a likable and talkative black woman, still living at the transitional shelter she had been placed in over a year before. She has no idea how long she has been there. This particular shelter takes in only elderly people and effectively operates as a sort of nursing home/boarding house. Josie has settled in, behaves as if this is her home and appears to have no plans to leave. However, her recall of the events that brought her there is scant and inaccurate in time frame.

Josie was born and raised in Tennessee and came to Chicago in her 20's to visit her uncle. After returning to Tennessee to get married, the first of three childless marriages, she came back to Chicago and married again. In her late 40's she purchased a large house with her mother and sister and lived there close to 30 years, first with family and more recently with friends. All of her family, except for two adopted daughters (who may be cousins) are deceased. She worked on and off throughout her life and was proud that she had recently attended a party for retired workers at the Drake hotel.

ES encountered Josie in the hospital after a burn accident in her home. She had been living in her house with a boyfriend of 8 years, Bob, who had reportedly been incarcerated for murder, another elderly white man (Joe), and later several younger residents, including alleged gang members, whom Josie does not recall. A neighbor lady occasionally visited and/or cooked for Josie and the elderly men. According to those who knew her, Josie's mental and physical condition declined considerably in recent years and she had started drinking heavily since meeting her boyfriend. Although she was not asked about her drinking she repeatedly denied such behavior during the interview. She had apparently lost her home due to delinquent taxes and was living there with no utilities in "deplorable conditions." The ES record noted that she owed over $2,000 to the gas and electric companies.

Over the next year, with followup from other agencies, ES twice removed Josie from her home (once after she wandered back there), placed her in the above mentioned shelter and secured a state guardian. According to ES and a neighbor, by the time she was removed from her home the second time Bob had died. Joe froze to death in the house shortly after her removal. Josie was obviously reticent about having to leave her home and frequently expressed concern for her possessions. She told us she left her home out of her own choice because she didn't want to live there by herself after "everyone had died" (implying that both Bob and Joe had died before she left). She feels that if someone "reliable" could have lived there with her, she would have stayed, but "when an old woman lives all alone people take advantage of you."

Currently Josie remains a long term resident at the shelter and she was unsure about the amount and whereabouts of her income. Shelter is no longer being paid by the City and the state guardian has been attempting to place her in a nursing home. Josie, however, likes the shelter and is attached to her "girls" there. She maintains for herself the image of having a home and a friend in her old neighborhood and talks about how she could visit. At the same time, Josie has been uncooperative in making nursing home plans, stating she is comfortable where she is. Despite her dependency and inability to maintain her life in the community, she struggles to maintain some sense of autonomy by refusing nursing home care, although she is essentially institutionalized in a shelter. She has coped with the crisis of being removed from her home by redirecting her attachments to shelter staff and believing that she still has her house and neighborhood, even though she knows she cannot return to it.

In Josie's case, some kind of institutionalization appears to be imminent. As we have noted before, this is not an uncommon outcome, especially for those who entered a homeless state in part due to dementia or other mental difficulties. An inability to cope, to effectively maintain (and remember) social networks and to manage daily (e.g., financial) affairs are characteristics of a number of elderly people who become homeless. However, not all those who become homeless are so vulnerable or so amenable to intervention by service providers. Those who are largely mentally intact and/or more resistant to service more often turn to their own informal social resources to regain housing.

For example, Lawrence Smith, a 72 year old divorced black man who is extremely frail, near blind but mentally intact, was evicted and homeless for a relatively brief period. Although ES secured shelter for him he refused to leave his south side neighborhood, stating he could stay with a friend, which he apparently did for a time. When interviewed, Lawrence denied that he has ever been evicted, saying that at the time he had already applied to CHA senior housing with the help of a friend and had left his prior apartment of his own accord. Despite his physical and financial vulnerability, Lawrence, and others like him, maintains a relatively independent and stable lifestyle with informal support. His pride and attachments to his friends and neighborhood preclude the need or desire to have formal service providers involved in his life.

Eleanor Jackson, an elderly black woman who never married is much like Lawrence in that she was able to rely on friends for assistance after she became homeless due to a fire. However, it took Eleanor much longer to find housing in part due to a weaker social support system and less organized mental capabilities (possibly mild dementia). She apparently alienated herself from many of those who helped her and was always hard to "keep up with." Eventually, after staying with a series of friends, she received formal help from a private agency in locating and moving to new housing.

Although many of the one time homeless come from fairly stable, long term housing backgrounds, this is not always the case. For instance, Margaret Scarola, a long divorced 70 year old woman, is strong headed, independent and healthy. She became temporarily homeless after leaving a boarding house where she felt she was being "poisoned." Despite her mental vulnerabilities and paranoia, Margaret was able to find housing in an SRO on her own after staying in a shelter until she got her next Social Security check. She has moved frequently, both in housing and jobs, and left several prior housing situations due to her recurrent fear of being poisoned.

Despite her transient lifestyle, her organized and somewhat overzealous approach to daily activities allowed her, for the most part, to secure new housing relatively quickly and easily. However, when confronted with questions about homelessness, Margaret seems terrified by the thought of having no place to go. She adamantly claims that "I'm not homeless myself—that's all I know!" If Margaret's mental state were to worsen and other factors were to change she could be at risk for repeated homelessness.

THE LONG TERM AND REPEATEDLY HOMELESS

The actual number of long term, chronically homeless "street people" represented in this study is relatively small, but their enormous needs and unique coping strategies deserve separate attention. Although we, and even the chronically undomiciled seniors themselves, may not know what precipitated the loss of a home, having already become long term homeless they are the most difficult to pull out of their homeless state. In one sense, they have adapted to life on the streets such that a neighborhood, a park or bench becomes their "home." Being attached to a lifestyle (albeit a harsh and difficult one), fear of institutionalization, and fear of being taken away from familiar surroundings are among some of the difficulties service providers must deal with when attempting to improve the situation of the chronically homeless. The following case description aptly illustrates how one woman's coping strategies are both admirable and frustrating to service providers.

Dana Kaczmarek: Avoiding "Intervention" While at "Home" on the Streets

Dana, 62 years old and of eastern European descent, has lived on the streets in the same neighborhood for at least 11 years. Numerous agencies and people in the neighborhood have approached her and tried to assist her in getting shelter, services and housing, yet Dana still lives on her bus bench and sleeps in doorways and nearby parks.

No one is certain how Dana came to be living on the streets. Apparently she never married but had two sons while in her early

30's. She lived with her parents until they died, when she was probably left with no income for several years. At least one son visits her occasionally at her bus bench and sometimes lives in the neighborhood. Dana believes that he will take her in, as he has made comments to that effect in the past. However, he is now divorced and agency contact with him and the other son has been minimal.

Although it is unclear just how she initially ended up here, Dana has clearly adapted to street life. She sleeps mostly in the day in regular places, occasionally showers in the park and dislikes shelters, using them only when it is very cold, preferring certain drop in and shelter services for women. She has been regularly turned away from a number of shelters due to her foul odor and incontinence. "Friends" on the street, where she is widely recognized, give her money which she "saves." She sometimes cooks in the park. She wears several layers of clothing, even in hot weather, and buys "new" used clothing every few months as she has no way of washing or storing it. Dana receives occasional food boxes from the local DHS office, meals at the local senior center, and is somewhat friendly with a few workers. Dana asserts, "I got everything I need in this neighborhood; it's convenient; stores are here; I go to the Diner or McDonalds. It's real nice outdoors. I like it here. I got sunshine." A rough tally of the resources Dana uses in the neighborhood reveals that her choice of this particular bus bench for a "home" is no accident. It is a rich environment, indeed. Some of the resources in her immediate neighborhood are mapped out in Figure 1.

Dana talks of getting a place or living with her son, yet she feels "I have enough money to live on outdoors, but not enough to live indoors. If I could find a sleeping room or a one room apartment I could live indoors. I don't want to get Public Aid or run up any bills." Dana is very unrealistic about the cost of housing and she does not want to pay more than $100 per month in rent.

Many agencies have been involved with Dana. Since 1983, ES has recorded at least 28 contacts with her, usually in winter when she presents herself to the local police station between midnight and 2 a.m. needing shelter. Agencies were usually unable to get beyond meeting her most immediate needs, and the ES record occasionally labeled her a "chronically undomiciled agency abuser" due to her

FIGURE 1

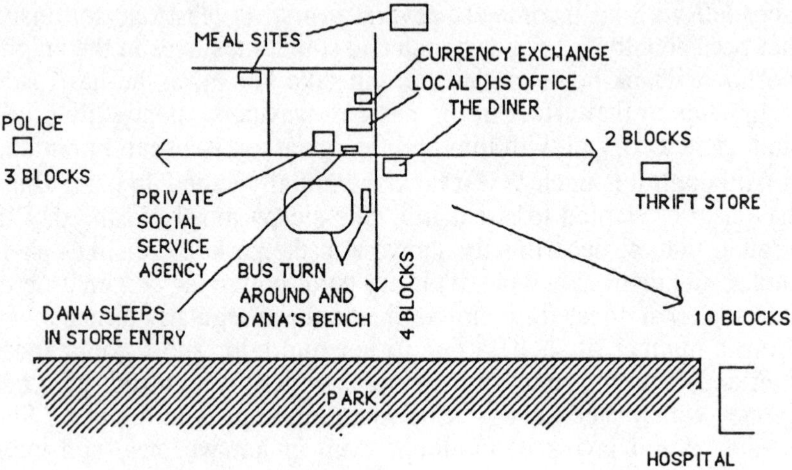

lack of cooperation. Health Care for the Homeless (HCH) occasionally houses Dana in a motel for a few days, but she gets fearful of "living alone" and sometimes leaves early. In the last year a state guardian has been appointed for her, a process which took a great deal of time and effort by Health Care for the Homeless. At the same time efforts were being made to put her in a nursing home. Dana herself refuses this and also does not want to live in senior housing which she perceives as being for old people. Currently, workers from HCH visit her regularly to monitor her health, manage her money and sometimes provide transportation to shelters. They initiated her $320 per month SSI checks and now dispense a weekly allowance to her. In the past they have arranged to pay for her meals at the Diner. "When her health starts to go, it will probably go fast, and we'll be there to facilitate what must be done."

In short, Dana, who has been diagnosed as paranoid schizophrenic and possibly slightly mentally retarded, maintains a life on the streets with limited social contacts although she admits to feeling "lonely." Some service providers (e.g., HCH) have established a moderately trustful relationship which assists her in maintaining her "home" on the streets, but she has not responded to more extensive interventions due to somewhat unrealistic expectations for housing, paranoia, and fear of institutionalization. Understandably, she refuses to leave the neighborhood she is attached to, in part because she is familiar with the informal and formal resources there and also because she is afraid her sons will not know where to locate her. Over the years Dana has developed effective coping strategies for survival which make it difficult, if not traumatic, to remove her from the streets.

A pattern of adaption to an urban "hunting and gathering" lifestyle is necessary among those who remain chronically homeless. After many years Dana and others like her appear to prefer this "unreasonable" choice. But the hardships and loneliness were evident in all the women we encountered who maintained the appearance of "bag ladies" and had histories of or exhibited symptoms of mental illness. Among the men we encountered, alcoholism was common. One such man, Reverend George Johnson, who died in a hospital at age 73 after a brief illness and stroke, had lived on the streets for eight years. He was described by his daughter as a "strong" and "determined" man who had "many homes" and for whom "life was exciting." According to his daughter, George's chronic homelessness began after the family

> . . . got burned out. From then on he left and went his separate way. We heard nothing from him at all for at least 8 months. He reappeared, but he must have gotten used to living on the streets by then. Apparently he thought that he had started the fire by his smoking or something.

George's wife and daughter had already asked him to leave since he repeatedly threatened to hurt the family.

George travelled the city daily with a large shopping bag of his belongings—"clothes, a radio, shaving kit, and his Bible and other personal stuff"—tapping into a wide array of informal social resources. He was friendly with the police who often lent him money. But he was a binge drinker who liked to show off his money. His daughter stated, "he lived for the first of the month. He would go to a whore house, get drunk on one beer and get rolled." He frequently talked violence as well, and was abusive. He was hard to live with, although his wife was always glad to see him, and he would have been difficult to help except on his terms. George's daughter felt that George probably preferred to die the way he did, hanging onto what he had, rather than to have ended up in a nursing home. Such chronically homeless individuals are making choices and asserting preferences among *very* limited alternatives.

A more common kind of coping pattern among the chronic and repeatedly homeless is that of being sometimes housed and sometimes homeless. Even Rev. Johnson was periodically housed by his relatives. We spoke with other men who, like George Johnson, have lived on the street and had problems with alcohol, but who expressed strong desires to find a place to live and in many cases, have done so. These individuals will often maintain a residence if given the opportunity and only fall into homelessness when evicted, for example, for drinking habits, psychiatric behaviors, mismanagement of finances, or temporary loss of income (e.g., due to being robbed). Such individuals may be better characterized as "sporadically housed" rather than "repeatedly homeless." The determination and self-organization required to pull themselves out of homelessness is substantial and not everyone can do it.

A vivid example of inability to cope with housing difficulties which resulted in repeated homelessness is evident in the case of Darlene Miller, a black 71 year old widow who has symptoms of paranoia. Darlene often lived with her dependent mentally retarded daughter which probably brought her an additional source of income in SSI checks. She had alienated her other daughter who she inappropriately believed to be the head of a gang. Darlene frequently ended up without a place to stay—being evicted, leaving apartments due to her fears and/or mismanaging her finances—either with or without her daughter. Since the early 1980's ES occasionally provided her shelter, a Reverend befriended and assisted her and other friends helped her on numerous occasions. Eventually she lived in a series of nursing homes interspersed with episodes of homelessness. Despite her difficulties and psychiatric vulnerability, Darlene repeatedly checked herself out of the nursing homes, trying to take charge of her situation and regain custody of her daughter. The nursing home she lived in at the time of the interview was one she had chosen with the assistance of a friend. Darlene was rather incapable of maintaining an independent housing situation, but nevertheless, in her own feeble yet sometimes effective way, kept trying to gain control over her and her daughter's lives.

COPING ABILITIES OF THE NEVER HOMELESS

The quantitative data (Chapter 3) has already shown that on average the never homeless had significantly larger monthly incomes, better social resources, better mental health and significantly less dementia (or other mental health problems) than those who had experienced homelessness. Despite these empirical differences, the overall "feel" of many housing situations of the ever and never homeless is sometimes remarkably similar. The potential of housing loss is widespread despite the fact that the never homeless are and have been in stable housing situations. It is the quality and context of these situations that are the really pivotal differences between them.

Three overall patterns of never homeless outcomes can be roughly discerned in the qualitative data. One is that some elderly individuals are so vulnerable (due, perhaps, to poor health or mental health) and so accepting of service that they come to the attention of the service network before homelessness is actually experienced. For example a woman confined to a wheelchair who had been living with her husband for many years in an apartment that was described as being in deplorable conditions came to the immediate attention of service providers when her husband had a stroke and died in the hospital. She was consequently hospitalized for malnutrition and did not resist eventual placement in a nursing home. Her dependency on her husband was effectively transferred to nursing home staff, despite the fact that she suffered some sense of loss and suspiciousness of the nursing home. Her plight was immediately recognized by the hospital which could quickly mobilize the other service agencies that were already somewhat involved.

A second pattern which emerges is that of individuals who are truly managing for themselves with adequate resources, having, for example, sufficient finances, active informal and/or formal supports and intact mental capabilities. Many of the SRO residents we interviewed fell into this category particularly if they can take advantage of the unique informal social resources available within that setting (see Chapter 8). We encountered numerous individuals who, although not necessarily assisted by family members, had received help from caring neighbors, landlords and otherwise invisible caregivers who sometimes take in near strangers. For example, Willie

Guenther, a single, 77 year old white man, lives with a family who befriended him after he was physically and financially abused by his girlfriend's sister several years before. When he was released from a hospital after treatment for malnutrition and dehydration, the Holts took him in and "nursed him back to health." ES encountered Willie after the Holts' son was arrested for drugs. The ES team tried to convince Willie that he was being financially exploited, but he refused service and continued to stay with the Holts. Despite the fact that he does not have control of his money, he seems happy there, enjoys playing grandpa to the Holts' younger children and has no plans to leave. Although Willie's coping abilities are not particularly strong on his own and he appears to have been dependent upon others and sometimes taken advantage of much of his adult life, he has chosen to be dependent on informal rather than on formal resources. In this case, his choice seems to have turned out relatively well and his situation appears to be stable. Without the Holts he would be at high risk, but the reciprocal advantages of their relationship and Willie's fixed income, make him quite secure.

Finally, an equally common pattern was that of individuals who were for a variety of reasons extremely resistant to service and had been able to get by on their own, although not always in the best of conditions. Within this category are also needy individuals at potential risk of slippage should, for instance, their mental capabilities change. Such persons often did not receive service even when they needed and wanted it. This latter category of the never homeless raises additional questions about the conditions under which some of these supposedly better off (i.e., not homeless) individuals live. The following represent two such cases: one man who refused service and one woman who would have been receptive to more help than she got.

Eugene Fuller: At Risk in His Own Home

Like Josie Hicks, Eugene Fuller, a 78 year old white man, had been living in his own home for over 15 years. He was living with his dog, in a middle income neighborhood when ES was called in to help "a senior living in deplorable conditions with no utilities." Unlike Josie, Eugene was effectively able to refuse services and maintain control over his decision to stay in his home. He was never placed in shelter and was never institutionalized.

Eugene had no children and got by with little assistance from those around him. His wife had died over six years ago and neighbors report that he kept their home immaculate, exactly as she left it, for some time. He later had a womanfriend, who had since disappeared, and he had a brother who was in minimal contact, both of whom he said stole from him.

About 4 years ago, neighbors began to notice changes around the house and a lack of care. Eugene became a "pack rat" and was increasingly "unable to take care of himself." The neighbors began bringing over food and eventually called ES for assistance. But unable to get him to accept any service. Eugene managed to subsist: he occasionally accepted food and minimal help from neighbors, he ran a generator in his garage for electricity (evidently because his utilities were disconnected), he collected cans for money, he bathed and washed dishes outside with the hose (possibly because of plumbing problems) and would let no one into his home. A neighbor reports that he received meals on wheels at one time, but that he was too proud to accept "charity." Eventually his health deteriorated and he became more vulnerable – he was hard of hearing, had arthritis and walked with a cane (which was stolen from him). Due to weakness (possibly malnutrition) and falls, he was in and out of hospitals.

In short, Eugene did not become homeless because he owned a home, had strong attachments to his house and the memory of his wife, probably had a decent income and lived a reclusive life, stubbornly refusing to let any agencies intervene. However, Eugene's living conditions had become unsafe and apparently unhealthy, complicated by medical and possible mental health problems. Though never homeless, he received little or no service, because he was "too proud" to accept help, and probably because he feared dependency on others and the possibility of being put in a nursing home. Even neighbors were able to provide him only minimal help. In the summer of 1988, he was hospitalized and treated for bronchitis, released to his brother, and only 3 days later he was hit by a car while picking up cans. Eugene died struggling to maintain his independence and his home while engaged in one of his survival strategies. Had he survived the accident, it is possible he would have been eventually removed from his house and placed in some kind of institutional care.

Viola Cooper: Alone in a Dreary and Dangerous Apartment

At similar risk, but so far experiencing a less unfortunate outcome, is Viola Cooper, a thin 70 year old black woman who continues to live alone in isolation in her basement apartment. She greeted us in the hallway with a toothless, pleasant smile. Her three room apartment, furnished with odd items of run down furniture, was cluttered, dirty and in poor condition: paint was peeling, pipes were exposed and leaking, and there were holes in the ceiling. This apartment, for which she pays $250 of her $490 monthly income, was not much of an improvement over the last apartment where ES had found her.

Viola's encounter with ES two years ago was due to a fire. She had just come home from the hospital after 8 days in intensive care for treatment of an infected bite on her face received from a rabid rat. She had been bitten while sleeping in her apartment. After the fire, ES determined that repairs on her apartment were "in process" and "relocation (was) not needed," although followup services record the deplorable conditions she was living in. After the fire, a new male tenant moved in next door, "a big dirty and greasy man who would not scrub out the bathtub," with whom she had to share the bathroom. When she complained, the landlord suggested that she move, "because I called the building inspectors and let them in." She tried to move. She found an apartment and paid the deposit and rent, but had no money left to move. Fortunately, she was referred by the City to a private agency which helped her move and gave her some furniture. Now, however, conditions at the new apartment aren't much better. She now lives too far from her old church to attend, for the first few months she had no running water or a working toilet, her only friend in this new building died a few months ago.

To us Viola presented a fine sense of humor and appeared to be a warm and tender person. Her apartment was decorated with hand written religious sayings and religious articles. She never had children, but had been married and had worked at a mental hospital for many years. This pleasant woman ended up in her situation in part due to health problems and loss of social supports in her old neighborhood. After a mastectomy in 1972, her husband of 30 years divorced her because "he didn't want to be responsible for the medical bills."

Currently Viola suffers a lot of pain and may have a recurrence of the cancer, although she has not had a medical exam in 8 years. She admits being lonely and depressed and her eyes watered when she talked about her desire to move into a "decent" place like a retirement center. She also said she wanted to work, babysitting or whatever.

In short, Viola has coped, being mentally intact and resourceful enough to locate another apartment and keep it. However, the quality of that housing is so poor and Viola so isolated that she is almost as vulnerable as the homeless. Alone, sick, and depressed, her condition is aggravated by the unhealthy conditions under which she lives (rats, leaky pipes and peeling paint). We could not help feeling that if she didn't find a more adequate and sociable living situation soon, she would probably not live long.

SOME OVERALL THEMES

Most of these cases describe individuals who are "difficult to reach" or in some way living on the fringe of generally accepted societal norms. Some exhibit reclusive behavior, suffer from alcoholism or diminished mental functioning or dementia, and some have never married or had children. Although we have not yet conducted systematic qualitative comparisons, we have identified some very general (and tentative) themes concerning coping capacities and housing difficulties.

Individuals experiencing a single, usually short term episode of homelessness exhibit two overall coping patterns: capacity to recover and regain their home or slippage into alternative paths of "pseudo homelessness" like institutionalization. Some individuals who come from relatively long term stable housing situations, like Lawrence, rather quickly resort to their own resources, including informal or formal social supports, to pull themselves out of what becomes a temporary crisis and thus regain stable housing. The period of recovery varies, depending on how much assistance individuals are able to muster or accept and how well they are able to manage their own affairs. Others like Margaret can display a housing pattern of instability (much like Darlene's) yet because they are independent and able to fend for themselves, can seek out new housing independently and still not end up on the streets, at least not permanently. Others, like Josie Hicks, are virtually incapable of maintaining adequate housing or caring for themselves, usually because of dementia or other mental problems or deficits. In most instances, at least with very old or frail people, a lack of coping abilities results in hospitalization and/or institutionalization.

In contrast, chronically homeless individuals illustrate capacity to implement creative survival strategies on the streets by maximizing available informal and "free" formal resources. The chronically homeless, contrary to popular belief, can display strong attachments to places, things (belongings) or people. At the same time, they may either enjoy or find necessary the freedoms of wandering and being outside. Certainly in comparison to the alternatives they fear, the threat of being put into a shelter, nursing home, or institution would deny such freedom. Thus some work very hard at avoiding that possibility. In many ways such individuals can establish a sense of "home" on the streets and maintain their privacy and autonomy by being "uncooperative" with agencies. At the same time the chronic homeless often experience alienation from family members and express desires to live somewhere.

Their abilities to maintain both informal and formal helping networks vary. For example, while George was able to maintain a fairly extensive part time informal network of relatives and friends to help him maintain his lifestyle, Dana expressed loneliness and wished she could spend more time with her sons. Dana, who was the most resistent to service, was most actively sought out for intervention, possibly because she was a timid, vulnerable looking white woman (Bachrach, 1988; Kutza, 1987; Rousseau, 1981). Those who appear to be chronically homeless in that they are repeatedly homeless, like Darlene, may lack some of the coping capacities and abilities to resist intervention that the street people have. Some may not live on the streets for such long periods of time in part because they have been less able or willing to cope with its rigors.

The cases of elderly individuals who were homeless are not always so different in general characteristics from those who were never homeless. In particular, Eugene's situation bears striking resemblance to Josie's except that agencies were unable to penetrate the wall of "uncooperativeness" and independence he struggled to maintain. Although both Josie and Eugene suffered from dementia, Eugene was better able to maintain his autonomy, possibly due to his better income, reclusive lifestyle, his learned skills of independence, and because he was a male. Viola, although she has remained housed, certainly lacks the amenities associated with having a "home." Ironically, Willie seems the least able to fend for himself, yet appears to have one of the better living situations by allowing his informal supports to develop and take over in a way that Eugene and others probably never could.

Whether homeless or not, most individuals' housing histories had been characterized by stability at some point in their adult lives, particularly those who were homeless only once or never. Even individuals living on the streets, such as Dana, might be characterized as having stable residences now because they have established regular neighborhood hangouts and routines. An outstanding theme contributing to instability or risk in individuals' housing histories is that of devastating loss: loss of a spouse or caregiver, a house, a job, income or services, or other basic necessities. If such losses are multiple and compounding, they profoundly disrupt an already vulnerable older person's environment. The nature and extent of such losses vary, but they are inextricably related with poverty and cognitive deficits.

CONCLUSION

If still living, virtually all of the elderly persons described above continue to live at substantial personal risk, whether or not they have been or are currently homeless or are in an acceptable living situation. Even if housed, the elderly can be living in a "near homeless" state, sheltered but with little quality, hope or meaning in their lives or their personal space.

Several of the persons discussed above struggled awkwardly but admirably to maintain their independence and avoid institutionalization and even hospitalization, by opting for the risks of poor health, poor housing and even death. While we can admire their autonomy and will, these are hardly "choices" people freely choose. That they take such risks indicates that for many individuals, true independence and autonomy of choice concern having a "home" as much as being sheltered. In cases where elderly individuals struggle to maintain their independence against all odds, it seems tragic that agencies and governments are unable to prevent traumatic situations such as the loss or deterioration of a home.

Without more analysis we hesitate to generalize about types of coping patterns. However, the varying coping abilities of individuals with housing difficulties within the context of other problems begins to suggest that there are certain coping patterns associated especially with the hard to reach elderly who are homeless or in deplorable housing conditions. For some, any crisis or change in the status of their resources can trigger a slippage into either one of these equally devastating states.

REFERENCES

Bachrach, L.L. (1987). Homeless women: A context for health planning. *Milbank Memorial Quarterly*, *65*: 371.

Cohen, C.I. & Sokolorsky, J. (1989). *Old men of the Bowery: Strategies for survival among the homeless*. New York: The Guilford Press.

Doolin, J. (1986). Planning for the special needs of the homeless elderly. *The Gerontologist*, 26(3):229-231.

Douglass, R. (1988). *Aged, alone & adrift*. Detroit: Detroit Area Agency on Aging.

Kutza, E. (1987). *Undomiciled elderly persons in Chicago*. Park Ridge: Retirement Research Foundation.

Rousseau, A.M. (1981). *Shopping bag ladies*. New York: The Pilgrim Press.

PART III: SRO HOTELS: A DISAPPEARING RESOURCE

Chapter 6

No Room in the Inn: The Disappearance of SRO Housing in the United States

Beverly Ovrebo
Meredith Minkler
Petra Liljestrand

SUMMARY. The relationship between the disappearance of the nation's SRO housing stock and the emergence of homelessness is examined. SRO's and their inhabitants are looked at historically,

---

Beverly Ovrebo, DrPH, is Associate Professor of Health Education, San Francisco State University. Meredith Minkler, DrPH, is Professor, Social and Administrative Health Sciences, School of Public Health, University of California at Berkeley. Petra Liljestrand, PhD, is Post-Doctoral Fellow, Alcohol Research Group, University of California at Berkeley.

The authors gratefully acknowledge Dr. Barbara Haley at the Department of Sociology, University of Maryland, and colleagues at the Institute for Health and Aging, University of California at San Francisco, for their assistance. This paper is based on research funded in part by the United States Administration of Aging, Grant No. 90-AP00003. The views expressed are those of the authors and should not be attributed to the Administration of Aging.

highlighting the demographic, political and economic trends which have shaped SRO housing policy over the last several decades. The argument is made that constructions of SRO residents as "deviant" and "undeserving" have resulted in public policy's failure to adequately confront the needs of this segment of society.

The epidemic rise of homelessness in the United States was fueled by another crisis—the disappearance of this nation's single room occupancy hotels ("SRO's"). This paper provides an historical look at SRO's and their inhabitants, highlighting the demographic, political and economic trends which have shaped SRO housing policy and reality over the last several decades. Notions of deserving and undeserving poor, and perceptions of SRO residents as deviant will be seen in part to explain the failure of public policy to adequately confront the needs of this largely invisible segment of society.

SRO's IN THE 1980's: AN OVERVIEW

Characterized by Erickson and Eckert (1977) " . . . as the cheap hotels and rooming houses located in areas adjacent to the downtown business district, . . . " (p. 440), SRO is an acronym for the Single Room Occupancy hotels in which large numbers of this nation's inner-city poor reside. As defined by the Department of Housing and Urban Development (HUD), SRO's are "partial rooms" lacking complete and private kitchen and/or plumbing facilities and housed within buildings of at least 12 similar units (Haley, Pearson and Hull, 1982). Viewed from one perspective, many of today's SRO's are private poorhouses and half-way houses supported by public funds (the majority of residents receive Social Security, SSI or Welfare), but without public accountability (Shapiro, 1971; Siegal, 1978). They provide specialized support for people unable to survive in the more open setting or society in general. The plethora of easily accessible goods and services available in city neighborhoods provide the daily living needs for SRO residents and are particularly important for the elderly and disabled who are most vulnerable to the demands of the SRO lifestyle (Cantor, 1979).

An alternative view is that SRO's are "the bottom rung of the housing ladder," the most affordable and least restricted form of housing available for those who cannot obtain other forms of housing, whether because of poverty and/or because of their being viewed as undesirable tenants for reasons including lack of references, poor rental history, disability, alcoholism or simply a "poor reputation."

For the most part, SRO hotels are old, cheap, and in deteriorating condition. The majority of SRO's in New York City were constructed in the last century. Ninety percent of San Francisco's were built before 1930, and the majority are not in compliance with current health, safety and building codes (Place, 1981). In Los Angeles, the majority of SRO's were built between 1900 and 1925 of unreinforced masonry, and thus face demolition since they are not in compliance with earthquake codes.

Although the rents for SRO's remain comparatively low, they are not 'cheap' housing for their residents and the majority of SRO residents pay well over the recommended 25 percent of their monthly income towards rent. Recent estimates for New York City suggest that the average SRO resident spends the equivalent of 73% of his or her total income on rent (Coalition for the Homeless, 1985).

Perhaps the most salient fact about SRO housing is that it has been deemed by HUD and other government agencies to be deficient and inferior and therefore until recently was ineligible for federal housing assistance. As will be noted later, even recent efforts to extend some federal programs to SRO housing have been too little, too late, and have coincided with an apparent phasing out of this type of housing stock.

Beginning in 1970, the number of SRO units declined precipitously. An estimated 1,111,000 SRO units were lost from 1970-1980 (Hopper and Hamberg, 1986). Many low income persons depend on this form of housing. Although the exact size of this population group is difficult to measure, research by Hull, Haley and Rothman (1980) suggests that in the early 1980's at least 1.7 million persons resided on a relatively permanent basis in some form of SRO living arrangement. While Hull et al.'s, definition is a broad one, including residents of boarding homes, apartments and private homes, their calculations suggest that fully three quarters of a million persons lived in the more narrowly defined "partial single rooms" in inner city SRO's.

Following a brief look at the history of hotels and the changing composition of the SRO population, current trends affecting the availability of this form of low income housing will be examined.

HISTORY OF HOTELS

The hotel as a housing and lodging form emerged in the 18th century, reaching its apex in the post-Civil War era, in response to an increasingly mobile, industrialized, and fluid society which required housing to be centrally located and to provide the occupant freedom from major household responsibilities. The hotel appealed to urban persons of all class backgrounds, both "social insiders" (wealthy and professional people, and young unmarried workers) and "social outsiders" (homeless men, migratory workers, prostitutes, alcoholics, etc. (Groth, 1983). The majority of current SRO's were constructed between 1890 and 1930. During the New Deal era and later, the shift in housing policy reflected a devaluation of hotel and apartment living, and a move toward suburban homeownership as reflecting mainstream American values, and as the proper and suitable housing form for the American nuclear family.

For urban Americans in the 40 years preceding the Great Depression, the hotel as a housing type represented urban living (high mobility and freedom) and emancipation, the latter especially for women, who were freed from cooking and other household duties (Gilman, 1904). During the Depression, options were closed off, and there was a retrenchment in dominant social values. The nuclear family and homelife were idealized, and transients and unmarried persons were characterized as irresponsible and socially deviant.

The years during the following World War II brought increased mechanization, and a decrease in the need for unskilled workers many of whom had resided in inexpensive, centrally located hotels. The change in the nature of manual labor affected the composition of inner-city dwellers, bringing a decline in the need for hotels as a primary housing source for a cheap labor force. This era also saw a flight from the city by middle and lower class families alike, many of whom received low interest FHA loans to buy their own homes. During the 1950's it was cheaper and easier to become a homeowner than to become a tenant. This coincided with a general increase in societal expectations, partly reflected in the federal commitment in the post-World War II era making possible homeownership for all Americans. The hotel came to represent housing at its most deviant and undesirable. Hotel residents were viewed as particularly irresponsible, epitomizing the general instability of tenants (Dreier, 1982). As hotels increasingly became seen as resting places for temporary guests, hotel residents were labeled transients. Finally, because hotel dwellers lived in single rooms, spurious assumptions were made that all were unmarried, and hence somehow threatening to the nuclear family and to the dominant notion which equated good citizenship with family membership. In the 1950's, a plethora of housing choices was available. Hotel dwellers increasingly came to be seen as persons who chose to be deviant by virtue of choosing hotel life, and who were by nature, therefore, irresponsible, transient, and not "family types." SRO residents were out of the mainstream of U.S. society, and hence not to be trusted, and were undeserving of assistance, recognition, or protection of rights.

In the 1960's, the traditional SRO hotel declined in numbers and in viability as a permanent form of housing. There emerged a new hotel type – the highrise – and along with this change occurred a transformation of the norm for hotel use. Whereas in the early half of this century, it was considered common for hotels to house permanent residents, the new highrise hotel housed almost exclusively tourists, traveling professionals, and conventioneers, accommodating in the process a new major industry – tourism. SRO hotels were relegated to a permanent second class status, desirable neither for permanent residents nor for transients. Furthermore, it became increasingly difficult to operate SRO hotels at a profit, since SRO's came to house the poorest of the poor by housing type. Buildings went without repair and renovation, and many of them had to be abandoned because of their dilapidated state. The populations which resided in SRO hotels during this period of decline included the cohort of destitute dwellers now aging with their hotels, plus a diverse group of urban destitutes, including ex-offenders, ex-mental patients, new waves of immigrants, and poor single persons of all ages.

The decline of the traditional hotel coincided with urban renewal programs of the 1950's to 1970's. Not only did the hotels deteriorate, but so did their neighborhoods, including the services and stores which made hotel living viable. Hotels were reduced to barely functionary structures, housing persons with many needs but provided with few options for meeting even the most basic demands of survival.

With gentrification during the last decade, American society has witnessed a return to the city. SRO hotels have increased in value, but it is the land the hotels occupy, not the buildings themselves, which are valuable. These forces in combination – the devaluation of hotels and hotel residents, the razing of urban neighborhoods in the Post World War II era, and gentrification – have created the current crisis for hotel residents and the hotels they occupy. And although the disappearance of hotels appears to be inevitable, no replacement housing is available or planned for displaced SRO residents (Ovrebo, 1986).

THE CHANGING COMPOSITION OF SRO POPULATIONS

The largest single group of SRO residents are the elderly poor. Research by Haley et al., (1982) has suggested a profile of the SRO elder as a white male with an average of 8.7 years of schooling and a total personal income of $4,410 in 1982, or 20 percent less than that of comparable non-SRO residents. The majority of elderly SRO residents had lived in their rooms for 5 or more years, and over half had never married. From 1976 to 1980, the elderly SRO population as a percent of the total SRO population increased from 62 percent to 69 percent. While this figure represented a *decrease* in absolute numbers from 191,000 to 183,000, as a consequence of the simultaneous reduction in the supply of SRO housing, it is nevertheless suggestive of the "graying" of a substantial portion of the SRO population.

In addition to the increase in the number of elderly persons competing for SRO housing, there has been an increase in ethnic minority populations seeking this type of housing. For example, SRO's in San Francisco's Tenderloin house 12,000-15,000 refugees from Vietnam in addition to thousands of Indo Chinese refugees from Laos, Cambodia, and Thailand. Los Angeles' SRO population, historically middle-aged or older single, white men, has been largely supplanted by homeless families, and young, single men of color.

The dramatic increase in the number of single person households in the United States over the past two decades also has had an impact on the demographic composition of the nation's SRO's. The 1980 census thus revealed 22% of households to be occupied by single persons in 1980, compared with only 15% in 1960. Low income members of this population group are not eligible for housing assistance unless handicapped, elderly or displaced. As such, there has been an increase in the numbers of low-income, able-bodies young single persons seeking SRO's (Kowal, 1976). Most of these individuals have had a history of social marginality and little choice in their housing options.

A final major subgroup within the broad category of SRO residents is the large number of ex-mental patients dependent on the existence of inner city accommodations. In the decade from 1965 to 1975 over 300,000 persons in the United States were discharged from psychiatric institutions. This development was the culmination of several events including the development of tranquilizers and anti-depressants, and legislation passed by Congress in 1963 to improve facilities for inmates making the transition to the community. SRO's were often the only available, affordable housing for ex-mental patients and deinstitutionalization thus added significantly to the number of unattached persons seeking inexpensive housing (Levine, 1979). In the mid 1970's, funds were cut for halfway houses and community mental health programs, forcing many more patients to move into SRO's. As Sokolovsky, Cohen, Berger and Geiger (1978) have noted:

> . . . in one year alone (1973-1974, 35,900 individuals were released from New York State psychiatric institutions and 14,580 of these persons returned to various environments of New York City . . . many have gone to live in one of the city's approximately 1000 SRO's . . . (p. 5)

The movement to humanize mental health care failed, due in part to the inadequacy of community mental health care (Bachrach, 1976). As a consequence, SROs became a revolving door for ex-mental patients, from the SRO to the city (acute receiving) hospital to the state (long-term chronic) hospital.

In sum, the 1980's witnessed a shift in the composition of low-income single persons seeking housing in inner-city areas. Where once this population consisted of white, male, unskilled laborers, it is now largely composed of the elderly, the disabled (including large numbers of ex-mental patients), young persons who are unemployed and/or socially marginal, ethnic minorities, recent immigrants (often living as a family in one room), and increasing numbers of women.

As will be seen below, these demographic shifts coupled with economic and policy developments, have contributed to a low income housing crisis which is intimately connected to the recently "discovered" problem of homelessness in the United States.

POLICY AND ECONOMIC TRENDS IN SRO HOUSING

The decreasing availability of low income SRO housing has been the combined result of housing policy decisions, urban renewal/downtown revitalization efforts and macro economic developments.

On the policy level, as noted earlier, perceptions of SRO's as "deficient" and their occupants as transients resulted until recently in the exclusion of SRO's from federal housing assistance. As one HUD official remarked in explaining his Department's reluctance to extend federal housing assistance to SRO's:

> We feel our obligation is not to subsidize or encourage the establishment of a housing environment which is in any way inferior in those standards of quality which our society has come to expect from the public as well as the private sector. (Werner and Bryson, 1982, p. 1000)

Indeed, rather than being the beneficiaries of federal housing programs, SRO's often have been the victims of these programs. While some recent efforts have been undertaken to correct this situations, they largely have been ineffective. The Omnibus Reconciliation Act of 1981 thus included a provision to make Section 8 moderate and substantial rehabilitation subsidies available to SRO's. Yet this policy change coincided with a reduction in Section 8 funds, and with what some analysts see as a phasing out of this program (Werner and Bryson, 1982). Between 1981 and 1986, the number of Section 8 subsidized units declined 76%. The Section 8 moderate rehabilitation program budget was reduced from $1.8 billion in 1981 to $133 million in 1989.

On the local level as well, recent efforts to provide housing assistance to SRO's not infrequently have had the reverse effect. In New York City, for example, a tax abatement ordinance to encourage the rehabilitation of deteriorated buildings was amended in 1976 to include SRO's. Ironically, however, the overall effect of the bill has been to the detriment of SRO's, with thousands of units being lost in Manhattan's Upper West Side over the past few years due to apartment and condominium conversions supported by this ordinance.

While the general trend in cities throughout the United States is toward an increase in the number of efficiency apartments, the number of elderly and poor residing in such apartments is decreasing. In short, the low-income elderly and unattached poor are being left behind by the conversion of SRO's to self-contained units.

Loss of Units/Urban Renewal. As noted earlier, SRO's are most commonly found in urban skid rows, inner-city commercial zones highly vulnerable to urban renewal (Erickson and Eckert, 1977). The federal government eliminated many skid row areas in the 1950's and 1960's. According to Lee (1978), in at least 41 cities, the skid row areas experienced net relative population losses of 38 percent in the 1950's and 30 percent in the 1960's.

Between 1960 and 1970, a continued dramatic decline in SRO housing stock was witnessed, representing a 16% decline nationally and an 18% decline in central cities. That drop is particularly significant when contrasted with the increase of all renter occupied housing units during the same period by as much as 14% in central cities (Hull et al., 1982).

These trends continued into the 1980's. New York City, for example, lost 89% of its SRO's and related lower priced hotel stock between 1970 and 1983 – a total of 113,000 rooms (Coalition for the Homeless, 1985). Seattle has lost fully half of its downtown housing since 1960, including an estimated 16,000 units of SRO housing (Werner and Bryson, 1982). San Francisco, while still proportionately the largest SRO center in the country, loses several hundred units each year, and lost 12,000 of its 31,000 SRO units between the years 1975 and 1982 (Paul, 1986). Denver's SRO hotels, which numbered only 45 in 1976, were reduced to only 19 in 1986. Predictions made in the 1970's that skid rows and SRO "grey ghettos" would no longer exist by the end of the 1980's, in short, proved to be surprisingly close to the mark.

During the 1970's and 1980's, the major forces behind the loss of SRO units were private commerce (downtown revitalization) and residential redevelopment (i.e., gentrification). Because federal funding has not been available for SROs, it has been economically unfeasible to rehabilitate old and deteriorating buildings. Those units lost since the mid-1970's have most frequently disappeared by way of abandonment, demolition or by virtue of having become uninhabitable (Haley et al., 1982). Conversion of SROs to apartments, condominiums, office space or tourist hotels has been the leading cause of the loss of units. In cities throughout the country, most notably San Francisco and New York, there have been numerous reports of illegal evictions of SRO residents, and of the cutting of essential services in order to facilitate conversion.

Economic Trends, SRO Depletion and Homelessness

As noted earlier, the past 20 years have seen joint trends of an increased valuation of SRO's for the land they occupy, coupled with a devaluation of the SRO building, the SRO lifestyle, and SRO residents. Inflation, particularly since the last 1960's, has exacerbated these trends. Because of their labor intensive nature, SRO operating costs have been rising at a rate faster than those of other types of housing. Those SRO's that survive are forced to cut services and raise rents, both of which make it difficult for poor people to live in them. In New York City, SRO rents increase with such frequency that the city now reports average rents on a daily, rather than a weekly or monthly basis. By 1984, these rates averaged $25-$35 per day (Coalition for the Homeless, 1985). Many SROs have been closed, torn down or converted during the past decade, and the neighborhood restaurants, stores and merchants that support the SRO population often are also forced to relocate.

The past decade has witnessed increased demand for SRO housing among the very poor at the same time that the supply of SRO units diminished. In many major cities, during the early 1980's, homeless correlated closely with the number of SRO units lost and the disappearance of SRO units was implicated by some investigators in the recent apparent increase in the numbers of homeless people in various metropolitan areas. For example, New York City reported 36,000 homeless in 1983, and a loss of 37,000 SRO units over the period 1975-1983 (Coalition for the Homeless, 1985).

With the recent wave of federal and local budget cutbacks, many essential social, health, and nutrition services for the inner-city poor have been sharply curtailed or eliminated altogether. Elderly persons and ex-mental patients are the SRO residents most affected by these cutbacks, and the diminution of services has been shown by some researchers to result in increased hospitalization, institutionalization, and even death. Since 1981, subsidized housing expenditures have suffered the deepest cuts of any social program. The total budget for the Department of Housing and Urban Development (HUD) was cut 78% between the years 1980 and 1988.

SRO's AND THE DESERVING/ UNDESERVING POOR

The housing trends and political economic developments examined in this paper help to explain the gradual disappearance of SRO's as a viable housing option in the United States. Yet the analysis of such trends is insufficient in its explanatory value unless accompanied by a consideration of the premises and assumptions underlying these developments.

Of particular importance in this regard is the notion of the deserving and undeserving poor, which lies as the base of much of our nation's public policy.

America's long history of concern with the deserving versus the undeserving poor has its roots in the British poor laws of the 1800's and has even been linked by some theorists (Williamson, 1982) to legislation dating back to the 12th century. That legislation provided differential relief depending upon the "deservingness" of the categories of poor in question, and began a tradition which continues into the 1980's. Preferential treatment thus is accorded low income widows (deserving poor) versus wives of deserted men (undeserving poor) and to low income Social Security recipients versus the poorer but less "deserving" recipients of Supplemental Security Income (SSI) who are stigmatized in the form and content of federal relief received. While detailed historical analyses of the concept of deserving and undeserving poor are available elsewhere (Ryan, 1982; Piven and Cloward, 1982) and are beyond the scope of this paper, the preoccupation of American policy makers with the notion of "deservingness" is relevant.

Nelson (1978) has elucidated this concern with respect to American services strategies for the aged, noting that most services policies favor the downwardly mobile aged, in part because they are thought of as "deserving and deprived," and further because they have become increasingly organized and able to press their demands on legislators. Service policies for the elderly hence tend to be "life enhancing," enlarging social opportunities etc., rather than the "life supportive services" needed by the aged poor. As Estes (1979) further has noted, "a major consequence of America's services policies is the perpetration of existing social class differences; they sustain stratification in that they do not alter the distribution of prestige, income or other critical resources . . . . " (p. 234)

The concept of life enhancing versus life supportive services has clear relevance to the field of federal housing assistance. By far the largest housing subsidies thus may be seen as "life enhancing" for the middle and upper classes, and involve a home mortgage tax deduction that cost the Treasury an estimated $42.8 billion in 1984 (Alter et al., 1984).

By contrast, life *supportive* services, in the form of housing assistance for many SRO residents and other low income groups, have been woefully inadequate. The rent voucher system of the Reagan administration, thus provides only about $200 million in vouchers to low income renters, and fails to reach many of the most impoverished SRO residents who fall through the holes of this particular "safety net." Ironically, moreover, the voucher system assumes the availability of large number of SRO's and other low income rental units at the same time that federal housing policy continues to contribute to their demise. One study estimated the shortage of low rent housing at 3.7 million units in 1985 (Center on Budget and Policy Priorities, 1989).

The changing composition of the SRO population from a sizable proportion of "social insiders" during the Post Civil War period (wealthy and professional people, and young single workers) to increasing proportions of less valued, social outsiders (e.g., unskilled laborers, the elderly poor, ex-mental patients and immigrants) has been accompanied over the last several decades by decreased federal and societal concern with the needs of renters. As noted earlier, a retrenchment in dominant social values and an idealization of nuclear family living from the Depression through the 1950's further underscored the deviance and undesirability of hotel dwellers and of the SRO lifestyle which they represented. Both the units and their inhabitants were viewed as undeserving and inferior and as such received inferior treatment and/or neglect in federal housing policy.

In recent decades, the rise of young urban professionals as a new and deserving population group has helped to spur the central city's growing numbers of high rises and condominiums. As noted earlier, such developments have been at the cost of hundreds of thousands of low income units, and effectively have displaced large numbers of less "deserving" central city residents, including, importantly, the low income residents of SROs.

Housing policies which have, at best, ignored and at worst hastened the destruction of SRO units in the United States have also reflected an underlying assumption that SROs because of their substandard nature, do not represent a viable housing choice. This assumption is a dangerous one, and further provides a rationale for the destruction of buildings which are not subsequently replaced by comparably priced units for displaced tenants.

The assumption that SROs do not represent a choice for their inhabitants overlooks the fact that such features of SRO environments as low rents, autonomy and centrality of location are viewed as desirable by some elderly and other tenants for whom the decision to adopt an SRO lifestyle is indeed a conscious and positive one.

The underlying assumptions that SROs and their inhabitants are deviant and undeserving, and that SROs do not represent a viable housing choice, in short, have combined to help shape housing policy which in turn has reflected these assumptions. The critical role of SRO's as the "bottom rung of the housing ladder" and often as an alternative to homelessness is, for the most part, neither appreciated nor acknowledged as the disappearance of SRO housing continues into the 1990's.

The SRO hotel as a generic type clearly is not suited to the wants and needs of a major segment of society, nor should SROs in their current, often dilapidated and overpriced state, be idealized. At the same time, these hotels remain an important alternative to homelessness, and it is not surprising that the rapid rise in homelessness coincided with the loss of the bottom rung of America's housing ladder. In the same way that homelessness has been "discovered" as a social problem, the disappearance of SRO hotels and the plight of their occupants needs to be brought to public awareness so that informed and comprehensive policy options can be developed and implemented.

REFERENCES

Alter, J. et al. (1984, January). "Homeless in America." *Newsweek*, 20-29.

Bachrach, L. (1976). "Deinstitutionalization: An analytical review and sociological perspective." Washington, D.C.: National Institute of Mental Health, Series D, No. 4, DHEW Pub. No. ADM 76-351.

Cantor, M. (1979). "The Informal support system of New York's inner-city elderly." *Ethnicity and Aging: Theory, Research and Policy*, by Donald Gelfand (ed). (New York: Springer Publishing Co., 1153-175.)

Center Budget and Policy Priorities, (1989). Report to U.S. Congress, Washington, D.C.

Coalition for the Homeless (1985). "SRO hotels: Standing in the way of the gentry." (New York: *Coalition for the Homeless and Tenants Rights Coalition*. Unpublished document.)

Cohen, C. & Sokolovsky, J. (1983). "Toward a concept of homelessness in aged men." *Journal of Gerontology*, 38, 87-89.

Dreier, P. (1982). "The status of tenants in the United States." *Social Problems*, 179-198.

Erickson, R. & Eckert, J. K. (1977). "The elderly poor in downtown San Diego hotels." *The Gerontologist*, 17, 440-446.

Estes, C. (1979). *The Aging Enterprise*. (San Francisco: Jossey Bass, 234.)

Groth, P. (1983). "Forbidden housing: The evolution and exclusion of hotels, boarding houses, rooming houses, and lodging houses in American cities, 1880-1930." (Unpublished dissertation, Berkeley, University of California.)

Gilman, C. (1904). "The passing of the home in great American cities." *Cosmopolitan*. Reprinted in *Heresies* (1981), 53-55.

Haley, B.A., Pearson, M. & Hull, D.A. (1982, September). "Primary individuals in single room occupancy (SRO) housing in metropolitan areas aged 20 to 61: 1976–1980." (Paper presented at the annual meeting of the American Sociological Association, San Francisco)

Hopper, K. & Hamberg, J. (1986). "The making of America's homeless: From skid row to new poor, 1945–1984." *Critical Perspectives on Housing* by R. Bratt, C. Hartman and A. Meyerson, (ed.) (Philadelphia: Temple University Press)

Hull, D., Haley, B. J. & Rothman, A. J. (1980). "Single room occupancy research study: State of the art report." Volume I. Draft. (Washington, D.C.: U.S. Department of Housing and Urban Development, Office of Policy Development and Research, Division of Housing Management and Special Users.)

Koenig, P. (1978, May 21). "The problems that can't be tranquilized." *New York Times Magazine*.

Kowal, C. (1976). "Housing needs of single persons: Will federal programs meet them?" *Journal of Housing*, 277-280.

Lee, B. (1978, September). "The disappearance of Skid Row: Some ecological evidence." (Paper presented at the annual meeting of the American Sociological Association, San Francisco, California.)

Levine, M. (1979). "Congress (and evaluators) ought to pay more attention to history." *American Journal of Community Psychology*, 7, 1-17.

Nelson, G. (1978). "Perspectives on social need and social services to the aged." (Unpublished paper. School of Social Welfare, University of California, Berkeley.)

Ovrebo, B. (1986). "A window on the world: Relationships between housing and health in a third class residential hotel." (Unpublished doctoral dissertation, School of Public Health, University of California, Berkeley.)

Paul, B. (1976, June). North of Market Planning Coalition, Personal communication.

Piven, F. F. & Cloward, R. A. (1982). *The New Class War: Reagan's Attack on the Welfare state and its Consequences*, (New York: Pantheon Books).

Place, D. M., (1981). "Residential hotel survey." (Sacramento, CA: Governor's Office of Planning and Research. Department of Housing and Community Development. Research and Policy Division.)

Ryan, W. (1982). *Equality*, (New York: Vintage Books).

Shapiro, J. (1971). "SRO as a village community." In *Communities of the Alone*, (New York: Association Press).

Siegal, H. (1978). *Outposts of the Forgotten*, (New Brunswick, New Jersey: Transaction Books).

Sokolovsky, J., Cohen, C., Berger D. & Geiger, J. (1978). "Personal networks of ex-mental patients in a Manhattan SRO hotel." *Human Organization*, 37, 5-15.

Werner, F. E. & Bryson, D.B. (1982). "A guide to the preservation and maintenance of single room occupancy (SRO) housing." Parts I-V. (Washington, D.C.: Clearinghouse Review, National Clearinghouse of Legal Services, 999-1009 and 1-25.)

Williamson, J. B. (1982, September). "Public policy and regulation of the elderly poor prior to the rise of the welfare state." (Paper presented at the Society for the Study of Social Problems and the American Sociological Association, San Francisco, California.)

Chapter 7

The Effects of a Shrinking Housing Resource on Older Communities in Chicago

Sharon M. Keigher

SUMMARY. A representative survey of SRO hotel conditions in Chicago, compared to Hoch's 1985 study, finds that the supply of this affordable housing resource has continued to erode. In the hotels studied, 10 to 30% of the residents are elderly. They tend to be long term and perceived as "desirable" residents. Pressures on certain neighborhoods with a high concentration of hotels are explored. A case study of a fire at one hotel reveals the "bumping" process through which residents become displaced.

Single Room Occupancy (SRO) hotels are one of the most affordable types of housing which has traditionally accommodated single inner city poor people. As noted in Chapter 6, the Department of Housing and Urban Development (HUD) describes SROs as "partial rooms" lacking complete and private kitchens and/or plumbing facilities and housed within buildings of at least 12 similar units (Haley, Pearson and Hull, 1982). Lawton and Hoover estimated in 1981 that approximately 130,000 (about .6% of) elderly heads of families live in hotels. About two-thirds of these were male and 88% were single. Hoch estimated in 1985 that Chicago had over 11,500 units of such housing and that approximately 10% of these were occupied by persons over age 65.

The author is especially grateful to Irene Gooden, Elizabeth Davy, and Dee Soustek who assisted with data collection at the hotels reported in this chapter, and to Donald Keigher for technical assistance, the owners and residents of the New Jackson Hotel for their openness and cooperation.

SRO housing in Chicago is limited and fragile, however. The Hoch study (1985) estimated that approximately 1,000 units of such housing were being lost per year due to conversions, demolitions, and gentrification. Such loss correlates strongly with the growth of homelessness all over the U.S. Kasinitz (1984, p. 10) shows that loss of SRO housing resulted from gentrification and that this erosion correlates directly with growth of the population living in shelters for the homeless. Baxter and Hopper (1981) and the Vera Institute of Justice (1981) both document the extent to which shelter users had been displaced from more established rooming houses and SROs. Rousseau (1981) notes that shopping bag ladies live intermittently in SRO hotels. Kasinitz notes (p. 11-12) how in city after city studies have confirmed how important SRO housing *used to be* to those who are now homeless, while Hoch and Slayton (1989) draw this conclusion very directly for Chicago. Erosion of SRO housing appears to have very direct consequences for poor elderly persons.

The SRO interview sample in the Chicago study was drawn primarily to be a comparison group of similarly situated poor persons living alone, since over 80% of the ES clients to be interviewed were living alone at the time of the emergency and about one-quarter were living in SROs or rooming houses. Because the supply of SROs is shrinking, SRO residents were assumed to be similar enough to the ES clients to have experienced similar threats to their housing stability. In the course of finding and interviewing this comparison sample of older SRO residents, we learned much about the importance and adequacy of SROs as a housing alternative for older Chicagoans.

Living in SRO hotels has been simultaneously underrated and romanticized. Depending on whose standard one uses, such settings might be viewed anywhere from "private poorhouses . . . without public accountability" (Douglass, 1988; Siegal, 1978) to something humane and exotic, the last great bastion of poor man's civility in a gentrifying city (Eckert, 1980; Ehrlich and Ehrlich, 1982; Lawton, 1980; Minkler & Ovrebo, 1985). Other settings, such as rooming houses and boarding houses, flop houses, missions and shelters are similarly at the bottom of the housing market and usually even less desirable alternatives by today's standards. They have older residents at least as poor as those in SROs, but such alternative housing arrangements have even more variable characteristics than SROs. Most are unlicensed, unregulated and consequently difficult to identify. The SRO hotels in Chicago, on the other hand, are easily identifiable because of special city licensing and code enforcement accountability and because of their need to maintain telephone listings and advertise. They present a fairly standard type of setting, at least for research purposes.

In the gerontological literature, SROs have been widely recognized as socially supportive, convenient and reasonably priced housing alternatives for seniors (Cohen and Sokolovsky, 1980). Ovrebo, Minkler and Liljestrand in Chapter 6 have noted that they are the most affordable and least restricted form of housing available to those who cannot obtain other forms because of poverty or because they are viewed as "undesirable tenants." Older residents acknowledge the benefits of hotels' locations near central parts of the city, convenience to services and amenities, privacy and social contacts. They are chosen in a free market by seniors of limited means who cannot or would not choose other alternatives in the marketplace.

SROs appear to sustain important informal helping networks (Hoch and Hemens, 1988) and social systems (Eckert, 1980; Smithers, 1985). They offer these strengths through an informal community highly respectful of personal privacy – apparently in ways different from formal housing complexes, organized retirement communities, trailer parks or public housing. In allowing and even facilitating natural social networks, informal help as well as accessibility to formal services, these informal systems both reflect and sustain an important part of the social organization of cities. Traditionally utilized by the seasonally unemployed, the addicted, and the mentally handicapped, as well as the elderly poor, and located in the downtown, skid row and red light districts, SROs have provided shelter as well as considerable tolerance for deviant individuals and activities. They are permissive and accepting of behavior disapproved by the larger society, while cleanliness, newness, and maintenance are less in evidence. Norms of respect for privacy and an assumption of autonomy continue to prevail. Community functions that take place in city streets, such as surveillance and emergency response, socialization of newcomers, and barter are critical (and yet only possible) in an environment so dense and visible, yet impersonal (Jacobs 1970). On the other hand, the "social organization" of such roles and communities is not always approved of by wider society (Hoch & Slayton, 1989; Cohen & Sokolovsky, 1989). It is based upon limited personal knowledge and a presumption of independence. This very freedom with its opportunity for personal choices is that which is typically denied by the regimentation inherent in long term care facilities today (Kane and Kane, 1989) and even board and care, and group homes. This freedom is precisely what old people fear losing if they have to relocate.

Finally, SROs play an important role for governments as an alternative to more structured, formalized, and expensive housing settings, especially in providing for the very limited, marginal or dependent in society. While SRO housing has been inadequately acknowledged as a resource, it has been widely exploited by governments in times of necessity, as in the dumping from state hospitals that occurred in the 1960s and 70s, and as contractual big city "welfare hotels" for homeless families in the 1980s. Today, with the reduced supply, SROs are playing an increasingly important role for cities faced with shortages of affordable housing, and to governments at all levels looking for market mechanisms to solve their problems. Governments charged with responding to such urgencies and constrained by severe economic limits can only hope for solutions offering decency. Differing city agencies, responsible for different problems and variously concerned with access, adequacy, or cost, struggle among each other to trade off their respective responsibilities for implementing certain functions (Hoch & Slayton, 1989; Kantor, 1988; Peterson, 1981). Production of housing stock and the imposition of standards of quality remain perplexing in the meeting of overall city needs.

RESEARCH OBJECTIVES

Given the current salience of low-income housing, an update of our understanding of the value of SRO housing to the elderly in Chicago is as valuable as the comparison of these elderly residents to the elderly who had experienced emergencies (presented in

Chapter 3). In doing so, this study started with valuable findings from Hoch's previous study.

Hoch (1985) studied 18 hotels selected to represent 115 low-rent SRO hotels in Chicago (of a universe of approximately 250). These were identified as buildings providing a 24 hour desk clerk or a switchboard at no extra charge, units with shared baths and units with kitchenettes. These represented 10,541 out of an estimated 12,500 units in the city. His data revealed that 10% of SRO residents were 65 years of age or older that 80% were male, and that 82% lived alone. While hotel residents tend to be more transient than other Americans, still half of Hoch's residents had lived there more than two years and 29% had lived there four years or more. Using this information as a base, our study sought trends and forces in the SROs that might be affecting the elderly. A second objective was to examine hotels in three specific locales where stock is threatened to identify older residents' options and preferences should this housing be destroyed.

A third objective, addressed in Chapter 8, was to describe older SRO residents' lifestyles and needs through the eyes of residents and managers, noting critical features of social and economic life in hotels that, if strengthened, would improve residents' access to needed services.

Sample Selection

The survey and interviews were conducted with hotel staff and residents at 27 hotels. The basic criteria for these contacts were to obtain enough information to select the senior resident interview sample, but also to provide a city-wide cross-sectional sample of hotels in which seniors live. Three areas were especially targeted for data collection because of the density of SROs there, including Uptown, the South Loop, and the area near the proposed stadium development on the Westside. In addition, however, it was important to have a sampling somewhat comparable to the Emergency Service sample, particularly in terms of race. For this reason, the Grand Boulevard area (Southside) was also targeted. Formal interviews were finally done in eight city neighborhoods.

Since the 18 hotels in the 1985 study were already a stratified representative sample, all but one were recontacted. However, full hotel assessments were conducted at only twelve because two were quite small, another would not permit female interviewers to enter, and three on the South Side were so "drug infested" or involved with criminal activity as to be too dangerous. (This area had presented difficult access problems in the 1985 study also.) Resident interviews in these areas were supplemented with interviews at the other hotels in these same neighborhoods.

In addition to these 18 hotels, 9 more hotel contacts were completed for a total of 27, allowing a broad view of currently operating SROs across the city. Three hotels where a feeling of stability and social support was particularly evident were studied in some depth. At these, in addition to the resident interviews described above, a short questionnaire was gathered from about 40 of the older residents. One of these hotels is in particular danger of closure because of city plans to redevelop the Westside Stadium area. Finally, in this chapter I describe the impact of a recent fire at another hotel to illustrate the insidious disappearance of housing resources and emergence of casualties.

SOME COMPARISONS OF FINDINGS WITH HOCH's 1985 STUDY OF SRO's

The 27 hotel contacts, together with the SRO resident interviews reveal a lot about the desirability of SROs as living environments for older people in Chicago, particularly the ways in which seniors and hotels cope with each other. Here we report on what appears to be happening to seniors as SRO housing becomes more difficult to find. We note the various pressures caused by certain neighborhood locations, rent increases, and the prevalence of seniors in certain hotels.

Seniors' Use of SROs as Scarcity Increases

Hoch noted in 1985 that only about 10% of SRO residents were age 65 or older. Based on our look at these same hotels, this overall proportion appears to be holding steady, although we found older residents somewhat clustered at certain hotels. In one-sixth of the hotels at least half of the residents were over 50, and in 40% of the hotels at least 25% of the residents were over 50. In our larger set of 27 hotels we found a slightly larger proportion of residents age 65 and over, ranging from 5 to 30% with an average of 17.8%, but this reflects our selection bias.

Older residents tend to be the long term ones. In the 1985 study half of the SRO residents had lived in their present hotel for two years or more, and 29% had lived there 4 years or more. In our sample, 86% of residents over age 50 had lived there two years or more and 76% had lived there four years or more. They had an average residence of 8.3 years at the present hotel and 27% had lived at their present hotel for 15 years or more! In a few cases these long term residents were also long term employees of the hotel. These older residents usually reported no plans or desires to move.

As a group, residents over 50 are relatively young. The mean age of the sample was 70, suggesting there are many pressures on older SRO residents that preclude them from moving to or remaining at SROs. In the period between ages 50 and 65, most residents apparently die or make some important decisions about relocating. Examination of residents' previous living arrangements suggests that it is not easy to find a room in another SRO, especially an affordable SRO in one's own neighborhood. If the previous residence was also an SRO, it usually no longer exists. While most residents had always lived alone, many had previously lived with their own parents or siblings, and others had previously lived with their children. The independence usually required to remain at an SRO, plus the attraction of lower rent in CHA (public senior housing) or other subsidized housing when one reaches age 60 appears to encourage a large proportion to leave.

Examination of the 18 hotels in the 1985 sample today confirms that study's projection that SRO housing in Chicago is disappearing. Between 1985 and 1988 one of these 18 hotels (one in the Grand Boulevard) area has closed. Two others in that same area have declined in quality to the point that drug trade and prostitution made them too dangerous for our interviewers to enter. (While such environments are obviously risky for older residents, some seniors do continue to live in these hotels.) Other areas have also experienced losses of hotels, most notably the South and West Loop areas, also many hotels in these areas have had rent increases that make them prohibitively expensive for persons on fixed incomes. While the proportion of rooms devoted to transient versus permanent rooms sometimes fluctuate, the number of rooms available per building seems to have remained about the same.

Rising Rents

The 1985 study noted that on average residents who paid by the month paid $161. Among these 18 hotels only three years later, we found rents ranging from $115-442 and averaging about $250. Of the 30 residents we interviewed, rents ranged from $160 to $366, with an average of $247. This rent level represents from 11 to 75% of the income of the residents we interviewed, with the average resident paying 47% of his income for rent. (The large range is due to the great variance in incomes since some residents are employed.) The three couples in this sample spend, on average, only 35% of their incomes for rent because of the economy of pooling their resources.

This 56% increase in hotel rents in the past three years, far in excess of inflation, is partly explained by the shrinking supply of SRO units which has increased demand. On the other hand, seniors tend to be long term renters and considered desirable tenants, so owners are likely to grant them a break or two. The rent increase for younger and newer residents has probably been even greater than for seniors.

There is substantial variation in rents paid by neighborhood. The South Loop rents are now particularly high as demolitions and gentrification creep into that area. Because of gentrification, many hotels there and on the Near North side, Near West, Greektown, and Lakeview areas no longer serve low income people at all. Even hotels which remain relatively inexpensive (under $220) have experienced rent increases of around 30%, which means that some of their previous tenants can no longer afford them. For example, we found only one resident over age 50 on General Assistance, which pays only $154 per month. He supplements his $170 rent by collecting bottles, although such earnings are technically illegal.

Price is not the only feature that might deter seniors from settling in SROs, however. Reduced supply and increased demand has meant that operators can be more selective of tenants. Marginally functioning and even disabled persons are somewhat less "desirable" than they were before.

Variation in Demographics and Prevalence of Seniors

One of the most lauded features of SRO living is that it naturally integrates persons with varying needs and characteristics, particularly on the basis of age and income. It is this mix and the informal barter that occurs naturally which strengthens the social setting (Hoch, 1985). Some operators, however, clearly prefer to have only employed residents, while at other hotels "naturally occurring retirement communities" have developed as seniors have remained in buildings with the right mix of amenities, rents and management attitudes. Often particular floors, and sometimes whole buildings, come to be occupied by seniors. While SROs continue to be occupied largely by men, women appear to be more likely to share a room than to rent one in their own names. Among the older residents, we found one in nine rooms occupied by a couple.

PROSPECTS: THREE SPECIFIC LOCALES WHERE STOCK IS THREATENED

Unique economic development pressures in three major areas of the city have served to reduce the availability of SROs in differing ways. These dynamic forces, complicated by other pressures reducing the supply of affordable housing, all have affected seniors.

Racially, the Uptown area is largely white, and prejudice and discrimination are evident in that several hotels still have no non-white residents. While most hotels are very run down and occupied by non-working, alcoholic or otherwise disabled residents, the edges of this neighborhood are gradually gentrifying. Many hotels specialize in some way, providing either board and care or an otherwise sheltered environment for the area's many residents with disabilities. (Uptown has been known since the mid-1960s as the neighborhood into which several Illinois state mental hospitals "dumped" patients.) Several hotels have direct agency contracts with area mental health programs to provide extra services.

The West Stadium area is mostly black, but Near West Side hotels are generally integrated. The neighborhood, including its hotels, is characterized by long term social networks with a palpable sense of community. Other hotels in the area are occupied largely by black working men. Even if hotels do not close, demand in this area will inevitably increase because of the loss of other low income housing in the area. The near West Side has already absorbed some pressure from the West Loop redevelopment of Presidential Towers and the razing of the last hotels on West Madison Street.

Finally, the South Loop area, which is the most racially mixed (typically white ethnic owners and mostly minority trade), and continues to have the most viable transient hotel trade, is changing the most rapidly. Closest to the most recently developed West Loop area and Presidential Towers, it appears to have absorbed the most SRO residents displaced from West Madison Street. Hotel rents in the South Loop are creeping up, and structural and cosmetic improvements are in evidence at many as they seek higher quality clientele. With a few strong exceptions, most hotels have mainly transient trade, and little sense of community. Ferns and brass have replaced the peeling paint in several first floor bars. A few notable exceptions are hotels in the way of large scale downtown development projects (including, ironically, the new Harold Washington city library) which have become visible nuisances. They are virtually empty and awaiting demolition. Gradually low-income people are being discouraged out of this area by rising rents, although a few older residents are being allowed "hold harmless" tenure.

Incidently, regional pressure was also found to have increased on the South Side around White Sox Park where the Illinois State Sports Facility Authority has bought the entire seven block area of South Armour Square. In the course of our research we stumbled upon the expedited relocation of this entire neighborhood with a population of about 600 people in single and multiple family homes. Most of the seniors were home owners who were offered market rates to sell. From talking with residents we estimated that about 100 potentially homeless single men who rented in that area would be displaced. By March 1989 the entire area had been razed and no agency any longer knows where the residents most vulnerable to homelessness have gone.

The human consequences of these forces are graphically illustrated by another, even more sudden crisis that occurred shortly after our research was completed, a fire.

THE ECOLOGY OF A FIRE: HOMELESSNESS IN PROGRESS

Seven months after our hotel interviews were completed, at 5 a.m. one chilly morning in March a three alarm fire seared through the New Jackson Hotel located in Greek Town. Like a giant game of bumper pool, first terror, then dislocation, and now permanent uncertainty has descended on a building that has been home to 108 residents for many years.

The Hotel

We had previously interviewed four men at this hotel, one that is remarkably racially and ethnically mixed. Half of the residents are over age 50 and most are men. Many are former skid row alcoholics, disabled to some degree, or on fixed incomes, and many have experienced homelessness at some time in the past.

A four story building, the hotel was built in three separate sections which have been breached and joined by rolling floors and meandering stairways. Built in about 1878, the New Jackson is believed to be the oldest continuously operating hotel in Chicago. The owners told us it used to house many vaudeville actors who worked downtown, and they have a 1900 vintage photograph of the original hotel from the Chicago Historical Society which they hoped to enlarge and hang in the lobby. The lobby, now decorated with faded technicolor murals of Florida beaches, is regularly occupied by about a half dozen men who hang around the front desk attendant and the bellman and their blaring little TV. Others sit outside on Jackson street on nice days, or tip a bottle in the adjacent parking lot, to the east of which is the Kennedy Expressway, and beyond this the downtown Loop. The front of the hotel at Jackson and Halsted Streets, is one of the busiest, most commercial, and most prosperous areas on the west side. Three businesses, a Greek fast food restaurant, a barber shop and a bar are on the Halsted side of the main floor of the hotel. Six blocks to the West is the proposed site of a new football stadium for the Chicago Bears. Two blocks to the South is the University of Illinois campus. The New Jackson, a strong and stable, but quiet community of low-income people, is in a classic location to be threatened by the very vitality and increasing affluence of its surrounding neighborhood.

The tenants here give new meaning to "long term" residence. A handful of rooms are for transients, but over half the residents have lived here longer than seven years, and at least fifteen residents are over age 65. Several employees live here. The hotel's maids have worked here 30 to 35 years. One bellman, who lived and worked here for 30 years, was recently hospitalized for lung cancer. Another started working here at age 17, and except for the time he was in the service, he has lived here for 50 years.

A Jewish family has owned the New Jackson since 1952 and day to day operation is managed by a father and son. Young Mr. Schlinn, who grew up in the hotel business, has a degree from Northwestern University and is now in his late 30s. Both men know many personal details about their residents and express genuine concern for their needs; while accepting of problems, they are intolerant of behavior that threatens other residents or property. They worry that the rent increases from $160 to $210 in the past 8 years now makes residence impossible for people on Public Aid, and difficult for Social Security recipients. Their daily presence at the hotel is partly required by the frailty of its infrastructure. They put a new roof on the building last summer, and recently replaced a boiler.

The Fire

The fire started in the third floor room of a transient guest in the west section of the hotel. We were told this resident was an alcoholic who smoked marijuana and that the fire started in a pile of debris near a wall in his room, although he was not there at the time. The official fire report said it was caused by faulty wiring. The fire spread quickly to the fourth floor and then into the ceiling area where it smoldered for quite some time destroying a major part of the roof. In addition to fire and smoke damage, the hotel sustained considerable water damage and damage to walls from chopping required to control the fire.

The entire hotel was evacuated and early news reports were that 70 persons had been displaced. One man was hospitalized briefly for smoke inhalation, but no other injuries were reported. Emergency service staff from the American Red Cross and the Department of Human Services (DHS) arrived on the scene and, because of the cold, arranged for two CTA buses in which the displaced persons could sit while relocation arrangements were made. Both Red Cross and DHS provided hot drinks, food, and blankets.

Processing of the fire victims took all day. Some from rooms that were less damaged were allowed to reenter the hotel and get a few belongings, which they carried out in shopping bags. Eventually the buses transported all the displaced residents to the Red Cross offices from which they were given food vouchers for McDonalds and shelter vouchers for two nights at local motels. By 6 p.m. 35 persons had been placed and the rest had been allowed to return to their rooms at the New Jackson. The 29 rooms in the damaged section of the building were all determined by the fire chief to be non-inhabitable and this area was closed off.

Thirty-three of the victims were placed at 5 different motels, three on the north side and two on the south. A DHS team took one 80 year old Hispanic man who "was pale and walked real real slow with a cane" to Walgreens to replace his medication and then placed him at a congregate care facility; another, a quiet old man with white hair refused to leave the area. He wanted to stay on a cot at the Red Cross building, but this was not allowed. He wandered away.

One man who was placed in a motel had just returned from the hospital the day before the fire. He was dependent upon two oxygen tanks and required the assistance of another man just to move around. Another motel placement was a man in his late 50s with only one leg who maneuvers on crutches.

The DHS Emergency Service list of the persons who were placed in paid accommodations that night is a cross-section typical of low-income housing. Eighty-five percent were men, 45% were black.

Ages ranged from 24 to 80, but tended to be in two groups: half were under 40 and 30% were age 60 or over. Twenty-five percent were listed as employed, but 20% had either no income or income only from Public Aid. Forty percent were on Social Security, either retired or disabled, and the rest were unemployed. The latter group included a 56 year old unemployed maid who had recently had foot surgery who shared her room with her 24 year old daughter and grandbaby.

In addition to those who were placed, several residents relocated themselves with friends or relatives. An Asian medical student who is soon to graduate anyway, will stay with friends. A couple of others, bothered by the commotion, decided to move out.

"Bumper Pool" Begins

On Monday morning when their vouchers ran out after two days, virtually all of the 33 displaced persons who had been in motels returned home to the New Jackson. At this point an intricate kind of bumping process began. A few transient rooms opened right away and were filled. A few other residents were accommodated in rooms that were gradually becoming vacant. The owners asked one unstable mentally ill young man to leave. He will live with relatives, at least for now. A woman in her late 50s, "who is kind of a packrat" and accumulates so much junk that her room is a fire hazard, was also asked to leave and her brother took her in. One man was arrested and jailed when the police caught him and a friend stealing TVs from the damaged section of the hotel. The owners asked the friend to move out as well. This shifting will gradually free up some rooms in the still open section of the hotel. The room of the mother and daughter sustained water damage to the ceiling and there was concern that the baby might eat the peeling paint, so they have placed the baby with other relatives.

At the request of the owners, DHS returned Monday afternoon to make "more permanent" temporary shelter arrangements for those the hotel still could not accommodate. Two more older residents were placed at the congregate care facility. In groups of 5 to 8 the rest were placed at various shelters for the homeless, with effort to locate places as nearby as possible. Discomfort with using overnight shelters was widely acknowledged. While several of these displaced persons have been homeless in the past, they are not "homeless types" now, but DHS policy disallows the placing of able bodied people at care facilities or paid permanent housing. Overnight shelters, however, do not permit people to remain in the building during the day; indeed most require that guests vacate by 6 or 7 a.m. and they are not allowed to return until 8 p.m. A placement worker was troubled when he observed, "Giving everyone paid shelter would be a problem for us because I just have a limited amount; I can't place everyone there. The guy in his late 50s, the amputee on crutches, had to go to an overnight shelter." A few days later, however, he got another room at the New Jackson.

The DHS coordinator visited the New Jackson five times in the week after the fire, and provided the owner with a useful directory of shelters and other social services. Each time a room opens up Mr. Schlinn gives priority to one of the shelter residents. A week after the fire, one of the older black men returned asking for his room back. He had paid up his rent through the next month and he felt he was owed a place to stay. Saying he would look for a room at another hotel, he was given a refund. It was noticed, however, that he needed the money now as he was broke. Most residents have let the owners keep their paid up rents with the hope that they can resecure another room soon. All of the staff are back now and Mr. Schlinn hopes to accommodate every one that has approached him for a room, at least "everyone we want back," in the next few weeks. A number are not coming back, however.

Prospects

A week after the fire, the damaged section of the hotel remained sealed off. Hotel staff were clearing out damaged carpet and debris. While the structure appears to be solid, the material and style of its construction cannot be replaced. Water damage to all floors and ceilings is extensive, as is damage to walls and ceilings where venting holes were made; crews are estimating the cost of replacing the entire roof and of cleaning up the business establishments on the first floor, so they can be reopened as soon as possible.

The owners indicate that the building has been "self-insured" ever since the insurance rates went so high that they had to make a choice between paying them or staying open. "Self-insured" means they have no insurance at all (but have to show proof of self insurability), which describes the situation of virtually all SRO hotels. Almost no one can get replacement insurance, or even liability insurance usually, because of the risks involved. "It's like trying to get medical insurance for a 90 year old man with a heart condition." And without insurance, they can't get loans for rehabilitating. It's a vicious downward cycle.

If repairs are made, each one will have to be financed from operating revenues and prioritized against the income producing capacity of the investment. The roof will be first, then the businesses, and hopefully the rooms. The owners could quickly be forced to raise rents. If its feasible, they definitely want to stay, but nothing is certain at the moment.

They could be forced to sell, but they are painfully aware that selling would be the end of this hotel. "No one looks at a building like this and says 'I want to buy an SRO.'" There is just not enough money in it. But many developers could become interested in this property, not for the value of the hotel but because of the obvious value of its location. There is a new Quality Inn just up the street. Plans for the West Stadium area have been publicized and private plans for the area are surely known to those who recognize opportunities. Information is worth money, and since this area is definitely scheduled to be redeveloped, information about it is presumably worth a *lot* of money. If the building is sold, "everyone" will make money, and there is surely strong community interest in improving the area.

One person we interviewed commented about the West Stadium area, "There will be more fires in the area. You watch the newspaper for the next year, that area especially, and see where the fires occur. There was another one not long ago . . . It's not really explainable, but things have a way of just happening. You see it in Uptown now too, on Kenmore Avenue, on the edges of the area as development moves in and poor people get crowded out."

Aside from the business and economic development interests of the many "big people" in the area, and the hotel itself, one question remains. What will happen to the residents deeply attached to this corner and this hotel? They have been coming back all week, and they will continue to come back, even if forced to stay at the shelters in the area as they are doing now. Why? This hotel is home. It is familiar and it represents the most meaningful attachment in most of their lives. It is also safe, and private, and so far it is cheap. It would be conservative to say that to many this hotel is life itself with everything that can be expected from it at this time. Besides being a tragedy for its residents, its loss would be wasteful to all the community. The city will continue to pay a terrible price for such housing loss until effective policies for preservation and creation of more low-income housing are adopted. Whatever happens next, the old timers at the New Jackson will probably be the last to know.

CONCLUSION

The disappearance of affordable and socially supportive SROs continues in Chicago as in other American cities because of pressures upon neighborhoods toward redevelopment and because of cities' complete lack of a strategy or incentives for preserving and improving them. The loss of this very valuable housing resource has contributed substantially to homelessness and unnecessary institutionalization of the elderly. The human terms of this loss will be illustrated in the next chapter as we explore the needs of older people which are met by SROs.

REFERENCES

Baxter, E. & Hopper, K. (1981). *Private lives, public spaces*. New York: Community Service Society.

Cohen, C.I. & Sokolovsky, J. (1980). Social engagement versus isolation: the cost of the aged in SRO hotels. *The Gerontologist*, *20* (1), 36-44.

Douglass, R. (1988). *Aged, alone and adrift*. Detroit Area Agency on Aging.

Ehrlich, P. & Ehrlich, I.F. (1982). SRO elderly: A distinct population in a viable housing alternative. In G. Lenoff-Caravaglia, *Aging and the human condition*. New York: Human Sciences Press.

Eckert, J.K. (1980). *The unseen elderly: A study of marginally subsistent hotel dwellers*. San Diego: The Campanile Press, San Diego State University.

Erickson & Eckert. (1977). The elderly poor in downtown San Diego hotels. *The Gerontologist*, *17* (5): 440-46.

Haley, B.A., Pearson, M. & Hull, D.A. (1982, September). *Primary individuals*

Chapter 8

How SRO Hotels Meet the Needs of Older Chicagoans

Sharon M. Keigher
Rebecca Hanson Berman

SUMMARY. Seniors living in SROs cite specific satisfactions and reasons for staying there, as do managers who prefer to keep them. Hotels offer a unique environment that usually requires maintenance of autonomy and the overcoming of structural barriers to accessibility, but can also facilitate vital and casual social interactions and some informal assistance. Social structures within hotels provide some important lessons for the design of social service delivery concerning convenience, reciprocity, meaning and attachment to people, place and way of life.

In one sense older residents of SROs are survivors who have remained here for some very specific reasons. This chapter explores what older SRO residents told us about their needs and about what is important in their daily lives – the essential reasons they continue to live in hotels. Most of them express little interest in relocating, and would not, except for the pressure just described in Chapter 7.

In Chapter 3 we noted that our sample of SRO residents has more resources than the sample of Emergency Service clients. Although SRO residents are somewhat younger, their relative "youth" does not explain this difference, and they generally are neither healthy nor wealthy. At least half of those over age 65 retired before their 65th birthdays, because of either disability, health problems or involuntary termination of employment. Several among the 50-65 age group are already retired non-voluntarily. Of all the SRO residents we surveyed, 17% are still working, 23% are disabled, and 57% are retired and receiving Social Security. At least 10% are working to supplement their fixed incomes while at least another 10% are receiving supplementary pensions or have some investment income.

At least 33% are also receiving veterans benefits, but typically only medical care.

In considering the needs and resources of such residents, we started by talking with hotel staffs, who had difficulty estimating residents' ages. (Desk clerks guessed at ages but rarely knew them exactly. Often the estimate of the proportion of residents over age 50 was quite different from the number of such persons that could actually be identified.) The estimates of need that follow, then, are "soft" data, simply reflecting staff's thoughts about what "older" residents need. Many positive dimensions of SRO living are identified, as are features of hotel living that could be enhanced further. Many resources available here involve the social milieu or feeling of community. By building upon such strengths and improving access to formal services, the quality of lives of older persons in SROs could be improved.

The following analysis discusses, first, reasons that hotel personnel mention for seeking or discouraging residence by older people, and then the reasons seniors give for living in hotels. We observed that the existence of long term casual relationships is overwhelmingly important in these choices. However, alleviation of physical barriers, access to formal services, and meeting of personal needs could certainly help seniors in hotels to "age in place" with greater ease and dignity.

WHY SRO MANAGERS SEEK (AND AVOID) SOME SENIOR RESIDENTS

Hotel managers varied impressions of older persons are revealed by their responses to questions about having them as tenants. Hotel staff members repeatedly told us that seniors are very desirable residents, because they have regular incomes, pay their rents on time, and are quieter and less troublesome than other residents. Indeed, several managers mentioned they would like to know advertising channels through which they could better reach potential senior tenants. These tended to be hotels that currently have unreliable tenants that they hope to evict, such as drug pushers, welfare mothers, and prostitutes. Some that "specialized," renting almost exclusively to seniors and offering reasonable rents, however, still felt they have difficulty reaching their market.

However, some hotels try to rent only to working people and do not seek or even want older residents. These include hotels "going upscale" and undertaking renovations, as well as those in working class neighborhoods where male residents all tend to work in the same industries. Others don't take "handicapped" people, sometimes because of building barriers, such as a few stairs or lack of an elevator that would exclude wheelchairs. More than one hotel manager observed, "We would like to take more seniors, but we can't modify the building to meet city standards." In a typical hotel, seniors are all on the fourth floor and the management is planning to move them all to the second because of fire regulations.

Other hotel staff noted, "We don't take mental cases" – usually because of some bad experience. Staff sometimes doesn't want people hanging around the building all day either, robbing, bothering, or frightening others. The greatest concern is expressed about "unpredictable" people who "might go off." The observant manager gets highly anxious if he feels that he has been left "holding the bag" by some agency that places a resident who is not stable. "If they function OK, I am willing to help, but I have some now who really don't belong on the streets."

The Saturday morning of our visit to one hotel there had been a dramatic incident. "This guy who was just out of the psych hospital went crazy. He apparently started shooting a gun out of his window or off the fire escape. He was manic depressive, about 40. He had only been here a week, had moved over here from (a men's hotel); he was too rowdy over there." An elevator full of cops had all gone up to get him, which created a lot of excitement.

Safety is a big concern. One hotel manager noted: "The neighborhood isn't really safe, especially for frail people, with gangs and crime and all. People hanging around are grown men, also kids . . . You wouldn't stand a chance if they took your purse." Another noted: "Older people are vulnerable to muggings in this neighborhood" (This small 40 unit building recently had a resident referred to as 'the stabber' who was arrested after murdering someone outside the front door.)

Finally, some of the more expensive hotels noted that, "Public Aid and SSI recipients couldn't afford to live here. After they pay rent ($260) they'd have only $60 or $70 left for food, and everything else."

Why and How Some Seniors Are Urged to Leave

A hotel might ask one or many older residents to move out for a wide variety of reasons. This occurs most frequently when the building is sold and the rents are raised. The new management, having no relationship with the "oldtimers," offers no special concessions for the difficulties a move would create for older tenants. Continuously operated hotels tend to give more consideration to long term residents.

Most SRO buildings have just a few elderly residents, ones that have resided there for even 20 to 30 years. These often are "characters," people that other residents tend to look out for. Some are reclusive and rarely leave the building, others are treated almost like "pets" by the management and other residents. Some have become the "institutional memory" of their neighborhood and their building, a repository of historical information. Most older residents, however, appear to contribute as much as they gain to the social fabric and sense of community of their building, such that their presence is valued even as their needs increase.

However, as they age some elderly residents may come to require too much daily care or monitoring. In other cases, incontinence, garbage accumulation, or pets might become insurmountable problems unless there is a personal caregiver who helps clean up. To the hotel, there is a danger of offending others in adjacent rooms. It appears that many hotels can easily manage one or two residents who require a lot of looking after, but if the building has too many elders needing care, the manager, maid and other residents may simply burn out.

The surest way to be evicted is failure to pay rent. (Many hotels guard against this by holding Social Security and other newly delivered checks at the desk, cashing them for free, and even securing residents' cash in the office safe.) Older residents without a fixed income or who cash their own checks, the very transient, and those without routines, are in greatest danger of eviction because of not paying rent on time.

Finally, those who irritate or bother the management, hotel staff, or other residents while offering no recompense run the risk of eviction if their needs become greater. These irritants might include things like misuse of hotel property, forgetting their keys, nakedness in the hallways, or abusing drugs or alcohol in public. Others are not likely to show consideration for persons who show no sign of reciprocating (see Smithers, 1985; and Hoch, 1985).

The procedure of eviction, while actually a legally prescribed one, is still effected quite efficiently by simply locking residents out or confiscating their belongings. Such measures are imposed usually when the rent is due and the tenant has already shown a tendency to not pay on time. While some operators admit having trouble enforcing rent payment schedules, most are very clear about their expectations and the sanctions they impose for lateness and non-payment. They are not in the business to run a charity, and all claim to have very fair rules which they enforce evenly. Several described having evicted people (rarely older residents, however) who then slept "out back near the alley" or in the back of a nearby bar where they got handouts, or otherwise "lived homeless" in the neighborhood for some time.

Clearly, then, having employment, good health, income, ability to protect oneself, lack of disabilities, and independence are all assets for an older person hoping to move into or remain in an SRO. And, in fact, most do appear to remain unless forced out by rising rents.

Why and How Seniors Remain in SROs Despite Increasing Needs

Why they stay. Our interviewers left a short survey at several hotels asking residents their ages and the reasons they chose to live at a hotel. Reasons most often noted include privacy and quiet, transportation and convenience, and affordable price. Others comment on the safety in the hotel, even if the outside neighborhood is not so safe. Most hotels go to a lot of trouble to secure the premises inside. Most are close to necessities, especially grocery stores, bars, and laundromats and a bus route which allows ease in getting downtown to the Loop. "Being left alone" and "the people are OK" are also mentioned. Obviously familiarity, habit and routine are terribly important to persons with limited mobility. Knowing the neighborhood, especially the merchants, friends, neighbors on the street and the neighbors in the building are also important.

Residents who have considered moving out usually mention that living in a Chicago Housing Authority (CHA) senior building would be cheaper. Those thinking about this option usually are not quite 60 years old yet, know that they will need to be on a waiting list for a long time, and several are on a waiting list already. Those interested are aware that CHA offers very affordable rent and a greater sense of security, especially in terms of personal safety. Several considering this also mention family members who have advised them to move either to retirement homes or to CHA.

Several emphatically said that they would *not* move "to no senior place." They do not like the idea of being surrounded by old people and of not being able to do exactly what they want, e.g., drinking, hanging out, or "watching the young ladies." Among those who do not move, there are strong feelings about reasons for not doing so.

How they stay. Most people over 60, even when poor and living alone, manage quite nicely without help in settings like SROs. This is the key reason most can remain, since many hotel managers share the feelings of one worker who said, "We treat everyone alike. It is a good building for seniors as long as they are able to care for themselves. Otherwise we don't have any special help available." Or, "They need to be independent, as no social and health services are available." Clearly, most older residents neither perceive they need services, nor use them, and hotel managers insist on this independence as a general rule.

Many times, however, we found that seniors remain as they get older, only because people in the building, management as well as residents, like them a lot and provide vital but incidental help. Long term residents as well as newcomers tend to "watch out for each other." Solid relationships have grown up over many years together through the familiarity and routine of day to day encounters. Helping out is convenient, as well as civil.

Occasionally meals on wheels or visiting nurses come in, but normally only when a resident has the resources to pay for this. Typically only well to do residents, or ones who qualify for Medicare-covered post-hospital assistance or some other special program, such as veterans benefits, are getting any formal services at all.

More often than not, staff in the building—the owner, manager or desk clerk, but also the maid, bell man, superintendent, custodian, or security guard—provide what assistance there is, helping out with everything from incidentals to personal care. In hotels that still have them, the maids are especially important in providing personal care, laundering clothing and bed linens, doing shopping and picking up carry out food, and cleaning floors, bathrooms, and cooking areas. Occasionally a maid does a great deal, though usually with extra compensation from the resident and only if she really likes the individual. The poorest hotels, however, provide neither maid service or linens.

The elder is also secure who has a "special" friend, usually a roommate, who will help out with personal care. Men tend to receive more help in this way, as lots of girlfriends help out even if they only visit intermittently.

Occasionally a resident is especially good at something and thus valued by the management. For example, one older white man was the plumber at a hotel with mostly black residents, although his vision was very poor and, according to others in the building, "he can't tell a nut from a bolt." This building has a new owner, lots of problems, and this plumber apparently knows every pipe in this very old building by heart. Another resident we heard of had such a "vile mouth" that whenever the lobby gets overcrowded or there is danger of a fight breaking out, the desk clerk asks her to come down. Her very presence as she talks to herself and rants at unseen voices is effective in quickly dispersing even a threatening crowd.

Since privacy and independence are such strong values here, another circumstance in which an elderly resident, even if quite sick, can manage to stay is one in which he or she insists upon staying. One is likely to stay who pays rent regularly and threatens a ruckus if the hotel tries to put him or her out. Even if others are extremely worried, residents are not usually "put out" unless management (and other residents, if they are involved) are satisfied that this resident really is willing to move. Hotel staff members sometimes affectionately describe many memorable residents who quietly remained to themselves, or had "come home from the hospital to die." Of a notable example, at one relatively well maintained, 40 unit racially mixed hotel, the researcher's field notes observe:

> One older black woman who was reclusive was found dead during the summer heat wave. She had been defecating on the floor, never took out her trash and was physically ill with emphysema. Her window could not be opened due to the way the phone in her room was hooked up, though the staff believed that, even if she could, she wouldn't have opened it anyway. Her body was apparently never claimed for burial. A nephew was contacted but did not want any involvement.

Such physical decline is a more regular occurrence at the larger hotels, and more often involves older alcoholic men with chronic untreated medical problems. A particularly observant owner describes his experiences:

> Well, a lot of residents don't take care of themselves. One guy would have lost part of his foot, but as it wound up, he lost his leg (because of gangrene). He had told me he was going to the hospital, but he wasn't. Finally I confronted him. When I lifted the sheet, his foot was literally rotting off . . .
>
> Then I had one of my employees who died here. They're just afraid, they've become so acclimated to a building, being on this corner, that they don't want to leave. And they are afraid of the outside world. So, even knowing they could run the risk of being very sick, even dying, they won't go to a doctor or a hospital or a nursing home. I've seen a lot of that over the years.

One SRO resident admitted her fear of medical care to us. This 79 year old woman, who looks at a hospital daily from her window, explained that the last time she went to the hospital, "They said something about cancer, that I have the kind like President Reagan has, colon cancer, but I ain't going to the hospital again." Later she mentioned a dear friend who had had diabetes. "She went to Cook County and she died there." Such residents need care *in place*, and often not very sophisticated care at all. This woman needs her toenails clipped and foot care, also a balanced meal once a day, and laundering of the bed linens – for starters. Her room also needs extermination for insects and vermin.

Others have a very real apprehension of being institutionalized. As one hotel owner described it, "I've seen a lot of my residents go to the hospital and never come back. They don't die, they just disappear." Not all go to nursing homes, either. He described two different residents that he later learned were virtually kept prisoners in what he considered deplorable unlicensed boarding houses. "Somebody got him out of the hospital and into this house on the South Side . . . There were three men in a little filthy room, kids running around, cockroaches everywhere, it looked like it should be condemned. They wouldn't allow them to use the phones, get dressed, or leave the building, or anything." Fears of such places, as well as of nursing homes, naturally discourage older residents from calling attention to their infirmities.

Clearly then fear, habit and routine, and lack of knowledge about how to get help and where to go explain residents' unwillingness to go to the hospital. Some hotels call upon the fire department and paramedics when such a situation reaches crisis proportions, but they usually do not. Many such residents simply need home care. Sometimes this might be formal care, but frequently it can be provided decently if not perfectly, by the people already around a hotel. The weekend desk clerk/custodian at one Uptown hotel described the kind of needs he sees:

> Mr. Smith has a nurse comes in once or twice a week. He is quite sick, has leukemia, and he's just back from the hospital. The maid feeds him every day. He is lonely. He also has a friend who seems to come in daily. People really like him, he is always glad to see you and very pleasant. His wife died just a couple of years ago, that's when he moved in here.

The hotel's structure and familiarity make providing such care and handling such situations integral to its routine and its life.

> Another guy died here last week. I had his pills. I often do that for people (take care of their pills), its just decency. He was just out of the hospital. The maid went to his room last week, but then when we didn't see him for a few days, we went up

and the guy was dead. So the police came, they sealed up the room.

On the other hand, the old age of the physical structures of hotels, their generally poor condition, and the great expense of building materials that are obsolete, make SROs challenging to maintain, at best. These structural problems present real deterrents to the elderly and disabled.

BUILDING FEATURES THAT COMPLICATE AND FACILITATE DAILY LIVING

Because SRO structures are so old, physical barriers like long or treacherous stairways, heavy doors, and poor lighting are simply taken for granted. Like other deterrents, we noticed that most of these impediments can be overcome if the residents and management choose to do so, but they are problems nonetheless. They gradually become problems for older residents.

For example, in one hotel with no elevator all seniors live on the 4th floor. One man with an artificial leg said he usually goes down only once a day, but he manages because others do errands for him. Another man, isolated and quite ill with arthritis, but whose hotel even has an elevator, emphasized the pain and difficulty he has going downstairs just to make a phone call or get groceries. "I have to get up, get dressed, and I'm really too weak to carry anything when I come back."

This "access to the outside" problem is often overcome with just a telephone, sometimes only a house phone. The desk clerk, typically at an antique switchboard, can serve as a life line, by calling certain residents every day and passively monitoring their activity. Unfortunately, telephone deregulation has made most PBX switchboards obsolete for making outside calls. Many hotels have had to remove the house phones from residents' rooms altogether or institute a charge of 50¢ or 75¢ for their use, creating a crucial deterrent for many residents. The phone companies have removed nearly all public telephones from the hallway floors. The man with arthritis told us the effort required keeps him from going to the lobby to use the only pay phone to call the VA Hospital, even when he is in a good deal of pain. Nor would he ask neighbors to perform so personal a task. The lobby phone certainly does not provide the privacy or comfort of the telephone he used to have beside his bed.

The old age of SROs creates another problem. Much of the old equipment does not work or requires continual maintenance and repair by a patient, skilled and preferably independently wealthy owner. Difficulties with roofs, boilers, gas lines, trash chutes, elevators, plumbing are constant. Many times such equipment appears to work, but on close inspection, does not. Elevators may be locked or require a bellman, or have doors too heavy for a frail person to push. At one Loop hotel the desk clerk noted, "If I had a penny for every time I open those doors for old people, I'd be rich." Ways are found to overcome such impediments, but they are real impediments, nonetheless.

The need for social contact, but also groceries and other necessities, are key reasons most older residents do leave the building regularly. Even the most disabled usually leave their rooms from time to time. Social contact is encouraged in hundreds of subtle ways by the hotel structure itself, with the decor and "attractiveness" of the lobby not necessarily being one of them. Most of the 27 hotels surveyed have a formal lobby or living room, but many show remarkably few signs of use. Those recently decorated, having new furniture and carpets, frequently have notices from the management nearby saying, "keep it clean," "Lobby for Guests Only," "Pick up your trash or we will have to close the lobby *again*. You know what happened last time." Even here hotel residents find ways to socialize.

The presence of a TV is a key indicator that the lobby is used and a clear message from the management that socialization is welcome. But we also saw many desk clerk's with little TV sets watching daytime soap operas. These also tend to draw an audience for specials, news coverage, and sports.

There is wide variation in the ways lobbies and frontage space is used. The cheapest hotels have all male residents and tend to be regimented, similar to a mission. One of these has about 30 chairs lined up in rows in front of the TV. The area clearly serves as a "living room" and the Tuesday we visited at two in the afternoon about ten men were watching a baseball game. Other places have threadbare but comfortable, overstuffed or barrel-type chairs against the walls or sometimes arranged in conversation groupings.

The higher rent places tend to have new carpeting of furniture; a good entrance seems to be the most important renovation to give the whole building a new look. With this usually comes signs about rules and admonitions about behavior. Most hotels have the lobby hours posted, usually closing at 9:00 or 10:00 p.m. Some of the buildings also indicated they had "curfews."

As Jane Jacobs (1961) notes, the presence of activity invites observers, and observers invite other casual observers, which basically makes an environment safe and interesting. Thus even "dead" space is important, as are sidewalks and other features in front of the building. Many such open spaces, however, provide no place to sit down, and "hanging out" is certainly easier for people with mobility problems if they have a place to sit. The important thing for socialization, however, seems to be the availability of space itself. Few hotels appear to have gone to any trouble to create sociable space and some evidently try to discourage it. Masonry structures with little sharp rocks sticking up to prevent sitting, or little points on the top of lead pipe railings and fences suggest that a manager at some time has gone to great lengths to control the use of such public space. Fortunately, socialization "just happens" anyway.

Along with available social space is the attractiveness and utility of other commercial establishments adjacent to the hotel lobby or on the street: bars, cafes and diners, beauty shops, laundermats, grocery stores, delicatessens, drug stores, and barber shops. Occasionally such establishments are owned by the hotel management. Besides convenience, such features provide important stimuli to people who enjoy watching and being a part of the community, even when their mobility and resources are limited.

In the poorest neighborhoods these assets include soup kitchens, food banks and shelters where persons can sleep if they can't pay the rent through the whole month. One manager in Uptown observed, "Checks come on the first and third of the month, that's when people pay and have money. By the end of the month several go on down the street to the Jesus People to eat."

The placement of windows in the building is most important for residents choosing either to be in and a part of the action, or to be left alone. One 70 year old man who has lived in the same room with "my woman" for 20 years appears to be greatly attached to the window by his bed. He sat comfortably there, slumped over with a cigarette, looking across the street. We met him out front where he spends most days "hanging out watching the girls" at the junior college across the street, usually while drinking corn whiskey. His interest in women is clearly articulated, "even though I cain't do nothing about it no more," and confirmed by the collection of nude female photos across the wall on his side of the room. (His mild mannered woman has poor eyesight.) Asked if he would consider moving to a senior CHA building he declared, "No. They wouldn't let me do this – hang out and watch the girls and drink. No way, I ain't going to no senior building."

Another man told us he really doesn't like it down at his end of the hall, "too quiet down here, never any action." This man also seems unaware that he is very hard of hearing. However, the darkness and lack of a view may be part of his real frustration. A 68 year old retired waiter, whose floor is covered with vodka bottles, has befriended a whole flock of pigeons which roost on his small once elegant window ledge. He has named several of the pigeons, including one "who is 'Boss,'" enjoys them immensely, and occasionally allows the baby pigeon to strut around his room. Unfortunately, some residents with a nice window and a busy view have the shade drawn all the time. Since they are usually at somewhat of a premium, it seems a shame to waste a good window on someone who doesn't enjoy and use it!

Many hotels place most of their permanent and senior residents on the same floors and in some places seniors are being moved to the second floor apparently in compliance with city code enforcement and to facilitate exit from the building in case of a fire. A secondary payoff might be the advantage Jane Jacobs describes, of having extra eyes and ears at the windows watching the neighborhood. Such surveillance makes the whole community a safer environment.

Besides the neighborhood itself, and how crime prone it might be, is the importance of safety measures within the building. At least some of this is reinforced by building features and procedures: bars on windows on lower floors, containment of traffic entering the front door which is monitored by the desk clerk for strangers, use of the telephone to obtain permission for entrance of guests, provision of quality locks on room doors, hallways set up to allow visual surveillance of cul-de-sacs. Even heavy traffic by familiar people in hallways provides assurance that one's door won't be tampered with.

Residents vary greatly in the arrangements of their rooms and belongings. Hotels vary enormously in the furnishings they provide and there is wide room for creativity in the things people do with a room all their own over a long period of time. A TV is usually the focal point for those who spend much time in their rooms.

Bathrooms can be a special problem for the very old, but rarely seem to be. Three-fourths of the residents we interviewed have a toilet in the room or share one with the room next door. Most rooms have a sink. Bathing facilities are usually located down the hall, however, and subject to hard use by many people. Bathtubs are generally difficult to step into, very dirty, and difficult for old people to bend over to clean. Showers were much more popular, and fortunately more prevalent.

Eating well is an activity immobile people have substantial difficulty with, yet again hotel arrangements can informally facilitate this through socialization and access to commodities. Rarely can residents afford to eat at restaurants, so creative ways are found to obtain groceries, store food, and pool resources. About half the units we saw provide a stove and refrigerator (which are usually very old and have maintenance problems, but some buildings rent out newer small refrigerators. The rest have no refrigeration, necessitating storage of food on window ledges in winter and disposal of left-overs in summer.

Hot plates appear to be disallowed at hotels on the Near North Side and sometimes in Uptown, but not elsewhere. Where they are utilized the management provides heavy electrical cords, and great care and concern is expressed about them as fire hazards. Both residents and management seem acutely aware of this, as well as the importance of being able to cook in one's room. Some very important social arrangements are sustained for years around grocery shopping and cooking. One of the nicest was a 62 year old amputee who regularly cooks in his room for an older man and a school teacher, and occasionally others. The teacher usually picks up the groceries and the two men pay the cook $1 per day. With this $14 he fixes breakfast and dinner for the three of them all week. When we met, he had just cleaned up from breakfast and was cooking chicken wings and soup for dinner.

Cooking and obtaining a decent diet is a substantial difficulty, however, for many. Many hotels are not located close enough to facilitate use of commodity programs, food banks, or senior meal sites or soup kitchens. Most residents, of necessity, plan their meals very carefully. Very few receive food stamps or any other government food commodities, although many have had them in the past. Many note that they cannot get to the office or stand in line for several hours anymore to apply.

The Inaccessibility of Formal Services

Use of formal social and health service agencies is relatively rare. Unusual is a 72 year old white man at a Near North hotel who receives meals on wheels and has two nurses visit daily from the VA Hospital. He is incontinent and non-ambulatory, but lives near the hospital. We met only one resident who utilized special transportation services which take him to appointments at Cook County Hospital for one dollar per ride. (Even the severely disabled resident with degenerative arthritis usually pays full cost to take a taxi.) Despite the poor health conditions of most of these residents, little evidence is seen of other health care service. Most residents know very little of services that are currently available and lack the money to buy them anyway.

A few hotels, especially in Uptown, seem to have arrangements with social service agencies which provide mental health services to targeted clients who reside there. Some agencies, such as Travelers and Immigrants Aid and Thresholds, place large numbers of clients and actually do regular group treatment at hotels. This is the exception, but seems to work relatively well.

Unmet Needs

In summary, the major unmet needs that are prevalent among SRO residents reflect their limited incomes and lack of information. Key deficits include: medical care, psychiatric care, and nutritional assistance. We have not here detailed the health care needs of this population, but a cursory glance indicates they are staggering, starting with basic needs for podiatric care, eye glasses and vision care, hearing aids, and especially dental care. Very few residents have enough teeth to really chew. Along with their real fears of hospitals and medical treatment is fear of change of any kind, including routines, and fear of strangers.

While hotel managers all express varying levels of discomfort with "crazy" or unpredictable behavior and usually with people who use drugs, a few hotels have worked out satisfactory arrangements with agencies to be placements in exchange for the agency providing back up services. While most hotels do not need the business this badly, more consultation and treatment would be helpful.

CONCLUSION

Hotel living is, by its nature, more likely to meet basic social needs than many other types of settings. Specialized assistance, though, especially medical and psychiatric care and basic durable medical equipment and supplies, cannot be provided easily and is badly needed by a substantial proportion of older SRO residents. Basic things like food, telephone, transportation are also needed, but most of these needs could be met by income supplementation and information.

Other services are identified by hotel owners and staff, but not necessarily by residents. These include actual service delivery, outreach, casefinding and case management. These services can be (and already are) delivered by neighbors and will be discussed in the last chapter.

REFERENCES

Hoch, C. (1985). *SROs: An Endangered species*. Chicago: Community Emergency Shelter Organization and Jewish Council on Urban Afairs.

Jacobs, J. (1961). *The death and life of great American cities*. New York: Vintage Books.

Smithers, J. (1985). *Determined survivors*. New Brunswick, NJ: Transaction Books.

PART IV: THE HUMAN COST

Chapter 9

The Needs of Older Persons at Risk of Housing Loss: Some Conclusions and Recommendations

Sharon M. Keigher
Rebecca Hanson Berman
Sadelle T. Greenblatt

SUMMARY. This chapter explores the implications of some of the earlier findings about elders at risk, especially the significance of social support, mental competence, and income. There is need for research exploring consumer perspectives and preferences, as well as agency constraints and flexibility. Services needed include health and mental health outreach, home maintenance and creative matching of natural helpers and formal care. Fundamentally, a national commitment is needed to "housing for all."

Little could be more basic to human identity, the quality of human life, and the civility of society than that every person have a home with decent and private personal space in which to live, rest and be reconstituted. Americans are clearly not guaranteed such basic provisions. For the elderly the loss of home and the security it provides is especially traumatic, and threats to such security are particularly worrisome. Losses leave scars not only on the immediate victims but also on communities. Thus, the especially human dimensions of housing and homelessness which we have highlighted here have special importance for *all* older people living in large cities.

Homelessness among the elderly is a very dynamic state, typically short-term and not repeated, but not always so, and disturbingly prevalent among certain vulnerable older populations in certain neighborhoods having certain endogenous and exogenous resources. Seeing homelessness and near-homelessness as a continuum of conditions rather than as a category allows us to focus not only on its immediate causes, but on the range of precarious situations which potentially lead to loss of a home and/or to institutionalization. Examination of the experiences of Emergency Service clients and SRO residents, as shown in Chapter 3, has revealed some statistically significant differences between the resources of the elderly who have been homeless and those who have simply been poorly housed. These critical differences suggest unmet needs that concern us greatly.

Second, and related to this, the problems associated with homelessness and near-homelessness have some distinctive characteristics among the elderly which are not found among younger populations. Some of these might be considered causes of homelessness, but many are conditions that simply exacerbate persons' vulnerability to loss of residence and autonomy in the community. Finally, careful assessment of the circumstances, feelings and lifestyles of vulnerable older persons have very important implications for the provision of assistance to them. Our analysis suggests important dimensions around which effective assistance must be organized and further research is needed.

DEFINING HOMELESSNESS

Our data has shown that homelessness among older people, while certainly not as prevalent as it is among younger people, has many of the same external causes: poverty, living in vulnerable neighborhoods and buildings, and attenuation of social support. However, homelessness as a descriptor does not adequately capture the range of venues by which the very poor elderly, a group we would expect to be vulnerable anyway, became dishoused. Homelessness is part of a process or a continuum of conditions resulting from a broad range of precarious situations. These are all relevant in a time of increasing shortages of low-income housing coupled with a society that is aging. As Boone and Weaver (1989) have noted, "more and more of the elderly will be at risk for becoming homeless and will exert enormous pressure on government to provide long-term care." Governments face a looming triple-jeopardy in attempting to adequately rehouse the homeless in general, care for a homeless population which is already "aging on the streets," and at the same time plan for growing future long-term care needs.

Nor is homelessness a permanent condition. When viewed retrospectively and longitudinally, individual cases of homelessness among old people are remarkably diverse and complex. Simply finding an old person on the streets or in a shelter does not mean that such a person is homeless, even though official city agents and surveyors often presume this. Street surveys of the homeless have highlighted a narrow band of situations and consequences and thus obscured a much wider range of at risky situations in which many elderly live. In a country which claims to provide adequately for its senior citizens, there is inherent significance in *any* elderly persons being homeless. The cases presented here illustrate the varied contexts that surround homelessness. The clients' own explanations of these situations illuminate how they could or could not have been prevented or resolved. Each of these individuals had coped in different ways; some were able to avoid homelessness on their own, others became its victims with or without help, and a few made the seemingly irrational choice to become or remain "chronically undomiciled."

Vulnerabilities of the Elderly to Homelessness

Examination of these data and comparison with other studies of homeless people confirm that the sample studied here is very broadly representative of the needs of older low-income Chicagoans and that living on the streets is relatively rare among this population. As a group, those who have experienced homelessness show some significant differences from those who have never been homeless.

The classic homeless "type," identified by Rossi et al., Sosin et al., Cohen and Sokolovsky (1983) and Douglass and in earlier years by Bogue (1963), and Bahr and Caplow (1973) are largely "young-old" single men, frequently dependent upon alcohol, somewhat disabled, but generally able to fend for themselves utilizing shelters and soup kitchens. Hoch notes that the increase in their visibility in Chicago is clearly related to the destruction of the West Loop and other skid row hotel areas and the continuing gentrification of certain neighborhoods. These men are most similar to the current residents we found in SROs who get few benefits or services. They sometimes deliberately evade social agencies and medical care. Many have had lives of transiency. Alcohol appears to play a bigger role in their transiency and homelessness than it does among younger populations. With increasing age these men come to the attention of outreach agencies which still have a difficult time settling them down, except in nursing homes. Many more float around in the overnight shelter system or staying outdoors, collecting cans and scavenging, passively moving on, rarely relating with others, and quietly dying of traumas or untended diseases. These marginally functional persons are more "exposed" now than in the past as the middle class has moved in on their neighborhoods and their previously cheap accommodations. Not seen as appropriate for the mental health system, they are "aging on the streets" nonetheless, and acquiring the additional physical, mental and social deficits that come with age.

There appears to be an increasing proportion of women joining this group, partly because they tend to live longer and have even fewer economic resources than men. These women are more likely to move in and out of residential settings. Society is less accepting of a transient lifestyle for women and these women apparently are less adapted to it than men. Such women are more visible to social agencies, more amenable to help and more vulnerable to violence.

However, when we examine the entire elderly population who have ever been homeless in our sample, both Emergency Service clients and SRO residents, much of this characterization becomes stereotypic rather than accurate. Homelessness is *much* more characterized by short term episodes than by chronicity. Typically the most vulnerable are those who live alone and whose locational or personal attachments are limited for a variety of reasons. They have typically experienced evictions for forgetting or refusing to pay rent due to dementia, the effects of alcohol, psychiatric problems, declining health or lack of trusted assistance.

These briefly homeless individuals are much like those in deplorable housing conditions if they move into an abandoned building, a rented room in a strange neighborhood, or any further isolating situation. More typically, those living alone in deplorable conditions are there for a very long time. The common risk of those without housing and those in deplorable housing is the vulnerability created by poverty, since low monthly income is more likely to be associated with inability to pay rent at all and to eviction. Similar risks are created by poor health and isolation for the two groups, but longevity in a place tends to make persons dependent upon and attached to their environment, especially as they begin to experience a decline in health or cognitive functioning (Rubenstein, 1989). This kind of deterioration is less risky for older persons in SROs, congregate housing, or communal neighborhoods where informal care and assistance is likely to be offered and accepted because personal relationships have been of long duration.

Homelessness is not the ultimate measure of poor quality of life. On average fewer of those in deplorable housing are receiving either informal or formal help than the homeless group, and they rate even lower on the total OARS scores. They are also less likely to be served more than once by ES or to be involved with other agencies of any kind. They typically lack the acquaintances found in the SROs. Despite being somewhat more likely to have children or other relatives involved, their situations are extremely difficult to deal with and guardianship is frequently recommended but difficult to establish, especially for those without relatives. Evidence suggests that agency inability or unwillingness to respond to the deterioration of such persons can have disastrous consequences. When forced to relocate by their social agencies, an eviction, or inability to pay rent, taxes or the mortgage on a house, the largest proportion of such clients go to nursing homes or places unknown. Of those who go to nursing homes, most do not live long.

Individuals who endure extreme losses or hardships in their elder years, sometimes prolonging life long patterns, sometimes seeking and sometimes evading the attention of the service networks, appear resigned to tragic consequences. It appears that many slip through the cracks in our service systems, but their disappearance is not necessarily the fault of formal service providers. A number of underlying factors help explain how such seniors end up in precarious situations and why, in many cases, services are not received until the situation reaches crisis proportions or, in some cases, never reach them at all.

The inevitable results of such trajectories are tragic, wasteful, and costly for society. For such persons, shelter is used to a surprising degree, usually as one of the most expedient resources available. Yet, shelter placement for a person highly attached to familiar surroundings is frighteningly disruptive. A colossal effort is required for return to normalcy, either at home or elsewhere. Effective but always tenuous relocations are made to public housing and in informal care through agencies, but regular monitoring is usually necessary to assure their ability. Any permanent settlement is almost inevitably made by a hospital, to another health care institution, involves public expense through Medicaid, and usually occurs when the client already has no other options or does not have long to live.

Clients who remain in deplorable housing conditions without consistent assistance die through trauma and accidents, acute and preventable illnesses, or through inevitable deterioration due to chronic conditions. Deterioration is expedited by the neglect.

Precipitating Factors in Homelessness Among the Elderly

In the face of a forced relocation, an elderly person must cope with the added hardship of declining health and functional capacity, fewer social supports, and sometimes diminishing economic and mental capacity. The combination of multiple resource deficits is clearly the most potent predictor of losing one's home. Loss of mental capacity is the most salient factor complicating inability to maintain surroundings, but loss of income, loss of financially supportive persons to share household expenses, and evictions are the clearest precipitants of homelessness. Without these predisposing factors and trigger events, the senior can frequently remain in deplorable, subminimal housing in a condition sometimes even more indecent than that of homelessness. The significance of these factors as precipitants to homelessness will be discussed separately in terms of our interviewed sample.

Aloneness and Lack of Social Support

A lack of social resources most clearly distinguishes the homeless from those who have never been homeless, but resources can be available in a variety of ways. Even when familiar and personal support systems have weakened, causal informal systems may be strong or have such a history as to continue to be helpful. Aloneness appear to be less of a factor for the elderly than it is with younger homeless populations. Many elders do live alone but have well developed coping capacities or receive substantial informal help. Indeed, life long aloneness (having never married or had children) may have actually produced more adaptability or resourcefulness. However, the loss of social support one depends upon, compounded with reclusive isolation, personal neglect, and/or depression or other mental problems is very serious, as is loss of any of the other resource for those whose reserve of social resources is already low. Such isolation is a critical factor in the situation of those in deplorable housing conditions.

Diminished Mental Functioning

Among elderly ES clients, diminished mental functioning resulting from loss of cognitive capacity, psychiatric disorders, and chronic alcohol abuse is the most prevalent corollary with need for service, affecting to 20 to 30% of our large ES sample (n = 475), especially the very old. This suggests that a substantial portion of the city's elderly are at risk and that, in the absence of other programs, city agencies (police, fire, and human services as well as aging programs) bear a large responsibility for their management. Fully half of the interviewees who were ever homeless and one-fourth of those in deplorable housing conditions present evidence of psychiatric or cognitive impairment. There is no question that cognitive deficits play a major role in situations that lead to homelessness among the elderly. Such homelessness is inherently different than that of younger populations.

Dementia is one condition with which society is normally sympathetic and provides attention through the service system, but if the client is also resistant, violent, or even simply passive, agencies which intervene often accomplish little. Behaviors that are a product of dementia – wandering, getting lost, and being unable to manage personal space and business – are common reasons seniors get referred to ES and other agencies.

Dementia is often confused with and compounded by psychiatric problems. Differential diagnosis between dementia, psychosis, and depression in the elderly is difficult for even trained specialists, so that we expected dementia to be noticed the most. Indeed, dementia is common in our large ES sample. Psychosis was less frequently mentioned in the ES records and in information obtained from others than was dementia. In contrast, however, among the housing risk sample (those homeless and in deplorable conditions), there was a substantial amount of psychiatric impairment mentioned while the most psychosis was seen among those who had ever been homeless, including the self-evicted and paranoid who took themselves to the police. This was significantly more than among any other group ($p = .009$). Despite this, the elderly in need of temporary shelter are much more likely to become institutionalized in nursing homes than in mental hospitals. Apparently the elderly are usually perceived as unable to benefit from psychiatric treatment and so are rarely admitted.

Very Low Income

A key distinction between the never and ever homeless is a relatively small amount of monthly income. On average the difference is only $161, the difference between $595 and $434, and the income for the currently homeless on whom we have information is much lower than this. With SRO rents averaging $250 it is easy to see why the margin for those who become homeless is simply too slim to secure or retain stable housing. This destitution is related to the fact that a substantial proportion of those interviewed have not applied for or are not receiving all the income and in-kind benefits to which they are theoretically entitled. This is largely due to lack of access and information: lack of transportation, telephone, and television; inability to read, fill out forms, follow directions and gather documentation; as well as inability to tolerate stress, lengthy bureaucratic processing and patronizing official behaviors, and to stand for long hours in lines.

CONCLUSIONS AND RECOMMENDATIONS

Providing Consistent and Basic Assistance

How can services be provided with a declining amount of low-income housing and a growing number of elderly people likely to experience housing related problems, including homelessness? In many ways it seems that service systems are being asked to do the impossible.

But still, assistance can be provided to housing risk clients that better meets their needs. Effective services must provide extra help and minimize risk, maintaining the equilibrium of current support systems (albeit fragile ones) while still supporting client autonomy. The key provisions must be preventive and early enough to deter both the loss of housing and premature institutionalization. The purpose of any such interventions should be fundamentally to listen carefully to the needs presented by seniors, both stated and implied, so as to respond to the ones they recognize. Thc bases of helping relationships are established by addressing their perceptions of what they need, and providing essentially what they want.

One key route through which this could be provided to high risk elderly persons is through provision of vital concrete services that people want and need where they live. The receipt of such service subtly obligates the client to relate and respond to the provider. Ideal for such purposes are provision of basic health care services and health monitoring which, given their lack of resources and fear of hospitals and medical personnel, this population desperately lacks. Provision of basic care such as toenail clipping, denture repair and prophylactic gum care, eye exams and provision of glasses, nutrition monitoring and provision of fresh and balanced food or meals, medication monitoring and regular refilling of prescriptions could not only encourage rapport and trust with the provider, but allow the opportunity for passive health monitoring. Health care specialists could follow and treat conditions such as hypertension, diabetes, cancer, alcoholism, metabolic disturbances, and heart conditions, the results of which are devastating, at the same time providing basic prophylactic care through regular visits.

Such care, however, is not unsophisticated, and psychiatric consultation needs to be part of it. An example is the Psychogeriatric Assessment and Treatment in City Housing (P.A.T.C.H.) program of Johns Hopkins University which operates in half of the senior housing complexes of the Baltimore Housing Authority (Tlasek et al., 1989). Approximately 13% of the residents in this housing authority are estimated to suffer cognitive impairment, and the program treats approximately 10% of the residents at each building. Responding to housing staff referrals, as well as self-referrals, the program provides consultation, casefinding, and treatment to chronically mentally ill residents suffering dementia, depression, and schizophrenia. By providing direct treatment consistently, it has deterred both evictions and unnecessary institutionalization. Providing direct benefits is a vital basis for beginning to win the trust of such clients.

In addition to health care, home repair and chore services to maintain the living quarters of frail elderly persons is similarly needed, whether elders' homes are owner occupied or rented. Situations ranging from the repairs of the New Jackson Hotel to restoration of Josie Hicks' home to the maintenance of Viola Cooper's apartment all require public subsidy of some sort to deter further deterioration and to guarantee access for poor people. Repair and chore services can assure that utilities are working, that broken windows are replaced, that vermin and burglars cannot get in. Unfortunately, it appears that "systems" of service, for fear of benefitting some gouging landlord, are more inclined to move old people from uninhabitable homes or leave them entirely to their own devices, than address the housing problem itself. Financing might be possible by placing a lien on the property or collecting the rents until the cost has been repaid. Correction of imminent danger and repair and reconnect of utilities and necessities is action which can effectively engender appreciation and cooperation from even the most resolute recluse, forming the basis of a helping relationship of strategic importance as the client continues to reside in this dwelling.

A second route through which important services could be provided would take lessons from daily life in SROs and neighborhoods with a strong sense of community. We know that autonomy is best facilitated with minimal assistance, and that sometimes quite complicated assistance is very effectively orchestrated through natural helping networks (Keigher, in press). We are reminded of a man we located in a South Side rooming house who had taken care of the old and dying alcoholic ES client in the room next door. The Department on Aging and Disability had sent out a homemaker, but she was allegedly attacked in the neighborhood and refused to go back. The caregiver said, "I carried him, I cut his hair, I cooked for him – and I got him looking pretty good, too. And I took him back and forth to the hospital . . . and nobody ever paid me nothing."

Aside from basic hands on care, the most basic kind of assistance is simply daily contact, surveillance and monitoring, attendance to needs, and accessing of resources. The key to effectiveness is the existence of a meaningful relationship and some sense of satisfaction for the caregiver. We can think of no more effective caregivers than the ones clients might choose for themselves, ones who are close by, easy to talk with, willing to help, matter of fact and likely to be already providing help. But such neighbors, relatives, friends and hotel staff have no obligation to help. If we want to sustain and promote assistance, as a society we need to provide incentives and reinforcement for doing so, providing a return that is meaningful to the caregiver, even when the client can no longer express gratitude. Reinforcement could take the form of rewards, recognition or financial compensation, but clients and caregivers should have choices in selecting these "reinforcers."

It seems reasonable to reward the informal caregiver for making a commitment to providing care for a set period of time. Given that hotel residents and staff are generally living below the poverty line, as are relatives and friends in poor neighborhoods, meaningful compensation levels need not be high in order to offer distinct incentives for the provision of such care. Such helpers can be of further value to agencies in doing case finding and outreach. Models for compensation programs are the Michigan Adult Home Help program (Keigher et al., 1988) and the VA Aid and Attendants Allowance program (Adamek, 1989). Each allow the client to select a caregiver of his or her choice who is paid a cash stipend based on a functional assessment of the clients' need. The maximum payment in the Michigan program is $333 per month.

Fundamentally, of course, funding for low-cost housing is imperative and none of these recommendations will be meaningful without it. Public support is necessary given the financial situation of those who have experienced homelessness, evictions, and most poor housing conditions. New units are needed, and some of such developments must provide supported care. Housing developments should recognize the importance of supportive housing and small group homes, places where natural helping relationships can develop and services can be provided with convenience, efficiency and non-intrusiveness. To assure such choice, some of such developments should be purposefully intergenerational. We must recognize that nursing homes are neither necessary, cost effective, nor humane for most low-income elderly persons (Kane and Kane, 1987) and certainly for most of the elderly we have described here as well. However, without permanent low-income housing, supported and facilitative of access to services, for most of these homeless elders the choice of a nursing home will be inevitable.

Finally, in the absence of indigenous helpers, formal agencies that provide home care services must be aware of the sensitivities, attitudes and prejudices of high need clients, and understand how significantly feelings and preferences affect clients' ability to accept services. There is need for appropriate assessment, flexibility in assigning helpers that are acceptable to the client, recognition of fears, and respect for privacy. It may be better to send no one rather than a helper who will discourage the client from seeking further help. Clients sometimes neither need or want the "service" that some agencies have available.

This is as relevant in crisis interventions as with any other need. A grave need exists to link up emergency services with followup services of other agencies that will continue to provide ongoing care. Too often emergency intervention provides a cataclysmic disruption but ameliorates very few basic needs. The magnitude of the immediate problem and need to respond quickly leads inevitably to a bureaucratic response: choice from a short list of short term options. The overwhelming problems presented by the housing risk clients we have identified make typical crisis responses quite inappropriate. Indeed, the basic problems are not emergencies at all, but chronic conditions generated by grossly inadequate resources (Lipsky & Smith, 1989). Besides provision of decent housing, food and medical care, ongoing casework and continuity in attention are fundamental.

Needs for Further Research

The findings reported above suggest two further areas of study that would improve our understanding of the housing risks of the elderly, as well as the capacity of our social service systems to respond to them. The first involves developing a more fine grained understanding of the behavior and needs of the kind of persons identified in the present study. Three categories of issues deserve further analysis, all having immediate relevance for improved design of social services. They include the following:

What is homelessness and housing risk from the point of view of the elderly person experiencing it? Such research would explore what constitutes "having a home" versus simply staying in a place; the meanings housing experiences have for the elderly. To further understand the perspectives of the elderly on homelessness (and whether this state is a valid or distinct category for them) we need to draw attention to what constitutes the range of alternatives in a continuum of the housed and the homeless (e.g., institutionalization, hospitalization, "subminimal" housing) and how these conditions affect the individuals experiencing them. An inherent issue within this framework is the importance of attachments – to places, people, memories, things, etc. An example of such analysis is Rubenstein's recent article (1989) on the meaning of home for the elderly.

What kinds of emergency shelter and other services are used by older adults and what does this mean to them? This issue not only suggests focusing on what is used but also when and under what conditions shelters and other services are not used. What are the kinds of nonuse and what explanations do the elderly give for refusing services?

Another category of analysis revolves around the interrelated issues of coping capacities, survival strategies and autonomy. In order to better serve the elderly at housing risk (both those needing relocation and those needing other services), we need to understand how some elderly people cope in the face of grave housing difficulties – how some survive and even maintain a degree of autonomy while being homeless, while others do not. Issues are deeply interconnected with:

- elders' explanations of how they survive (whether homeless or at risk) and their descriptions of the loose collection of information and/or formal resources they turn to,
- their perceptions of their life and lifestyle focusing on issues of fantasy, denial, privacy, independence and fear,
- internal intervening factors which appear to play a part in their housing risks and/or their ability to accept services, such as alcoholism, dementia, mental illness, fearfulness, reclusiveness, and dependency conflicts,
- external intervening factors which impact upon housing risk and service use, including abuse, neglect or estrangement from others, deteriorating health, loss (financial, social and otherwise), support of dependents, etc.

A holistic, in-context examination of the situations of elderly individuals along such dimensions may reveal elderly types or categories of at risk individuals prone to slip into homelessness or other equally unhealthy conditions. This would allow a more careful and judicious targeting of preventive and interventive efforts by emergency as well as case management services.

The second area of research that is needed would draw upon the first, but would focus on agencies and how they are coping, given the apparent unresolvability of problems presented by many high need clients. For example, starting with the randomly selected sample of housing risk clients in this study, systematic research would examine these clients' sources of formal help and the utility of such help from the clients' as well as agencies' point of view. By looking "from the bottom up" at the system of services, research would identify agencies in the emergency service and aging network and examine how each typically responds to elders in crisis. It would examine stated procedures and policies, as well as actual practices. Agency "responsiveness" would be explored regarding how elderly persons get into the emergency service system and beyond. The study would acknowledge agencies' perceptions of elderly clients and their definitions of need, beginning to identify agency flexibility and what could be more creative packaging of services, addressing the costs of treating basic social problems as emergencies (Lipsky and Smith, 1989).

In conclusion, we must state unequivocally our conviction that all the diagnostic resources, client service, and research in the world is not going to alleviate the growing crisis in urban housing which is threatening America's elders, as well as families, children and working people in the prime of their lives. According to the National Housing Task Force (1988), from 1974 to 1987 the number of households with incomes under $5,000 (in 1986 dollars) grew from 2.7 million to 4.7 million. Yet, in that same period our nation's production of federally subsidized HUD housing dropped on average from 167,000 units per year to less than 25,000, an 80% drop in the past decade. This erosion is compounded by the potential loss of more than one million more units of federally assisted housing through the termination of low-income restrictions or the expiration of subsidy contracts. And current production efforts offer little hope of increasing the supply of low-income units in the near future. A sizable and growing proportion of our population is underhoused, unhoused, or living in uninhabitable conditions.

Until our nation adopts a federal policy and commitment to "housing for all," development patterns of American cities are going to continue to force those with limited resources and marginal housing into homelessness. The cost to all agencies of "servicing" such persons—of outreaching, case managing, arresting, "guarding," following up, crisis intervening, band aiding, institutionalizing and intensive caring—appears to be far greater than that of simply housing them decently in the first place (Lipsky and Smith). The many services we have described here, that have been demonstrated and proven effective over and over, do not work in the absence of a decent and affordable home.

REFERENCES

Adamek, M. (1989, March). *Caregiver views of cash assistance as a support for in-home care*. [a study of the V.A. Aid and Attendants Allowance program.] Paper presented at Conference on Family Care: Research and Policy Agendas for the 1990s, Michigan State University.

Bahr, H.M. & Caplow, T. (1973). *Old men drunk and sober*. New York: New York University Press.

Bogue, D. (1963). *Skid row in American cities*. Chicago: The University of Chicago Press.

Boone, M. & Weaver, T., Eds. (1989). The changing face of homelessness in America: Part one. *Practicing Anthropology*, *11* (1).

Cohen, C.I. & Sokolovsky, J. (1983). "Toward a concept of homelessness in aged men." *Journal of Gerontology*, *38* (1), 87-89.

Douglass, R. (1988). *Aged, alone and adrift*. Detroit Area Agency on Aging.

Kane, R. and Kane, R. (1987). *Long-Term Care: Principles, Programs and Policies*. New York: Springer.

Keigher, S., Simon-Rusinowitz, L., Linsk, N. & Osterbusch, S. (1988). Payments to Informal versus Formal Home Care Providers: Policy divergence affecting the elderly and their families in Michigan and Illinois. *Journal of Applied Gerontology*, 7(4), 456-473.

Keigher, S. (in press). Informal supportive housing for elders: A key for preventing self-neglect. *Journal of Elder Abuse and Neglect*, *3*(2).

Lipsky, M. & Smith, S.R. (1989). When Social Problems Are Treated as Emergencies. *Social Service Review*, *63*(1), 5-25.

National Housing Task Force (1988, March). *A decent place to live*. Washington, DC: National Housing Task Force.

Rossi, P., Fisher, G. & Willis, G. (1986). *The condition of the homeless of Chicago*. Chicago: National Opinion Research Center.

Rubenstein, R.L. (1989). The home environment of older people: A description of the psychosocial processes linking person to place. *Journal of Gerontology: Social Sciences*, *44* (4), S45-53.

Sosin, M.R., Colson, P. & Grossman, S. (1988, June). *Homelessness in Chicago*. Chicago: School of Social Service Administration, The University of Chicago and Chicago Community Trust.

Tlasek, M., Robbins, B., Roca, R., & Storer, D. (1989, March). *P.A.T.C.H. Psychogeriatric Assessment and Treatment in City Housing*. Paper presented at Conference on Family Care: Research and Policy Agendas for the 1990s, Michigan State University.

Appendix: Methodological Notes on the Chicago Study

Sharon M. Keigher
Rebecca Hanson Berman

SUMMARY. This appendix details the deign and methodological approach utilized in the Chicago study. The methods focused the study on individualized housing risks as well as the city's interventions. Discussion of data collection describes the sample selection criteria and procedures, sources of data on both ES clients and SRO residents, interviewer procedures, and the processes of locating the selected clients. It concludes with discussion of data management and qualitative analytic methods utilized.

This study has blended both quantitative and qualitative methods in its approach, utilizing a data source that was believed to provide a unique but comprehensive view of the varied needs of Chicago's seniors. In contrast to "street survey" methods of identifying the homeless, it relied on client records to identify those "at risk" and to provide clues regarding the causes of homelessness. While it certainly includes a substantial share of persons who have experienced homelessness, it does not find great numbers of long term or currently homeless people, nor does it focus exclusively on the problems of the latter groups.

The authors acknowledge the assistance and guidance provided by Madelyn Iris in the design of the qualitative research methods reported here.

POSSIBLE METHODOLOGICAL APPROACHES FOR SUCH A STUDY

Sosin and associates note (p. 20) that "Nearly every study of the homeless faces a most difficult definitional decision about the nature of the group to be described." Much of the confusion over the actual magnitude of homelessness has arisen because of differing approaches to counting them derived from these differing definitions of homelessness. Rossi and associates, for example, sampled only from preselected census tracts determined to be frequented by homeless persons and only sampled those persons literally sleeping on the streets, in abandoned buildings, and in public from 1:00 a.m. to 6:00 a.m. who had no place to go. His study also counted persons sleeping in shelters. See Douglass (1988) for an annotated bibliography of studies of homelessness including comments on methodology.

Sosin and associates' study, however, used a wider sampling frame to survey persons who were likely to be living "doubled up," in treatment programs, or otherwise not paying rent. His researchers interviewed people at the places where they were most likely to go for necessities or to obtain services, such as food pantries and shelters. He mentions a third type of homelessness which his survey could not include, short term homeless persons and families housed by agencies in motels or with vendored providers, who are scattered across the city. "To some, this group may be homeless; to others it may not be (p. 21)." He estimates that this group would be relatively small on any given night, but because they are served by a variety of public and private agencies, this group's experience has important implications for policy making.

The present study has a special interest in this third type of population, especially in terms of what the public sector does for this group. The sampling frame in the present study includes data from agency case records on clients who have been vendored, as well as persons (the majority) who have received no such assistance nor even had a need for shelter. The approach used here has an additional advantage in that it incorporates interview data as well as agency case records. The Kutza (1987) study cited above is an example of a case record review, but it included no interviews. The present study does both, and supplements this with further information gathered from other agencies, as well as friends, and neighbors familiar with the client.

DATA COLLECTION

Research Schedule

A pilot study of City records of emergency services to the elderly was conducted by the principal investigator in the summer of 1987 with support of a Gerontological Society Fellowship, sponsored by the DAD. The research study reported in this volume built upon the pilot study and was conducted from June 20, 1988 through Feb. 15, 1989. The research schedule is outlined in detail below.

Summer of 1987	ES sample of 125 drawn.
June 20 to August 10, 1988	Additional sample drawn and descriptive data from agency records collected.
June-July, Sept-Oct, 1988	Survey of SRO hotels.
June to July, 1988	Interview instrument developed and tested.
Aug 1 to Dec 18, 1988	SRO resident interviews conducted.
Aug 1 to Dec 18,1988	ES interviews conducted.
Nov 1 to Feb 15, 1988	Analysis and write up.

More time than originally intended was spent in negotiations with city officials to secure access to their files, in developing and testing the assessment instrument and in locating some elderly ES clients, thus delaying data analysis by two months from the schedule. The followup contacts originally planned for all selected clients were made impossible by these delays. However, much followup information was gathered by research staff who continued to receive calls from agencies, friends, relatives and neighbors throughout the fall, even after data analysis was being conducted. In some instances more than one visit was made with the client. Consequently, however, complete data is not available on every client who was located.

SAMPLES

The ES Sample

Emergency Services are delivered in the following way. After initial screening in the telecommunication center at DHS to determine if an emergency actually exists, ES teams are dispatched by car to respond to calls for help from all sources, but especially from police, fire, social agencies, neighbors and citizens. These teams complete a contact card for each situation they investigate which is then filed. The files consist of 55 drawers, each containing an average of 864 cases. Approximately 11% of these are blue cards which designate clients aged 60 or older. Therefore, sampling consisted of picking four-digit random numbers, the first two digits designating the drawer and the last three digits designating the number of the blue card within the drawer. If the drawer did not have as many cards as the number drawn, that number was discarded. In this way, each card had an equal chance of being drawn.

However, since the ES team is charged with dealing with the immediate emergency and referring the individual elsewhere for any further help needed, the data gathered at an initial contact is minimal, serving only to deal with the problem of the moment. Names, ages, sex or race are not always recorded. More explicit identifying information (i.e., social security numbers, last known address, names of family members) is less likely to be recorded. As a result, the files contain some records with the same name, but often nothing to indicate whether or not these are the same individuals. The sample is therefore not ideal, but within the limitations placed by an operating program that is concerned only with single interventions, the sampling process has not added to any biases that may already exist in the agency records. There is no reason to suspect that systematic biases exist that would invalidate our conclusions.

From a universe larger than 47,500 client contact records from 1984 to 1988, two samples were utilized. The first, drawn in the summer of 1987, consisted of 125 cases of clients over the age of 60 where the last recorded emergency occurred any time before July 1987. In June of 1988, a second sample of 475 senior cases was randomly drawn from all ES records (approximately 9.2% of the estimated 5200 elders in the file at that time). From this set of 475 cases, four types of seniors were identified: clients who had no record of housing related crises; those who had a record of having been in need of temporary housing or shelter or had been evicted; those whose record indicated substandard housing conditions; and those where there was recorded both poor housing conditions and the need for temporary shelter. Cases where fire had been recorded, but no effort had been made to arrange shelter, were included in the first type. The second, third, and fourth types were considered "housing risk cases." Comparisons made between these four types are generalizable to the full aged client population of the ES program.

A sub sample of 115 cases (including 123 clients – 6 couples and 2 pairs of sisters), was identified and selected for interview. This was a purposive sample, chosen for having had housing related crises and recent enough contact with the agency to have a strong probability of being able to locate and contact them. These 115 cases included both housing conditions and shelter need clients. Fifty-five came from the new (1988) random sample of 475, specifically from the subset of housing risk clients whose last contact with ES had occurred in the past year and would be easier to locate. Sixty were housing risk clients from the original pilot sample drawn in 1987 (Keigher 1987) whose last contact was anywhere from 1 to 4 years previous to the research and thus presumed to be more difficult to locate.

This sample was designed to permit the comparison of characteristics of older persons in a variety of risky housing situations: the undomiciled; those in their own homes; and those in a variety of other types of housing. Eventually we located and obtained in-depth information on 91 of these 115 cases. But, the interviewed sample is no longer a random sample from the files of housing crisis cases.

The SRO Sample

SROs studied were drawn from a sample used in a previous University of Illinois study of Chicago SRO housing conducted three years previous to this research (Hoch, 1985). This city wide weighted sample of 18 hotels were of varying sizes when interviews were conducted previously. This was ideal for replication because of its representativeness. Investigators from our study contacted all 18 of these same hotels, but could only complete assessments on 12 of them. Fifteen more hotels were surveyed in areas where neighborhoods (including SRO's) are determined to be on the verge of gentrification and redevelopment or are already undergoing transition. This added to our sample 6 other hotels in Uptown, 1 in the West Stadium area and 7 in the South Loop. The total sample of 27 hotels represented the following six priority geographic areas: (1) Uptown-Edgewater-Lakeview, (2) North Loop, (3) South Loop, (4) West Side near the proposed Bears Stadium, (5) Westown-Humboldt Park-Logan Square, and (6) Grand Boulevard-Kenwood-Oakland.

In addition to the characteristics of the hotels, the characteristics and preferences of the older residents were studied. A sample of 30 residents aged 50 and over living in 12 selected SROs were identified and interviewed to obtain equivalent demographic data for comparison purposes. A sample both older and younger than age 65 where chosen in order to compare the importance of social security and other entitlements in personal choices. With an estimate of the number of seniors in each hotel, interviewees were chosen on site at each hotel by selecting every 11th room from a list of all residents over age 50 in the hotel developed by the hotel manager or desk clerk. Where a couple lived in the room, they were usually interviewed together.

In fact, however, the selection of older residents was partially determined on the basis of who was home and willing to be interviewed. Elderly who worked or were otherwise out or busy during the day were less likely to be interviewed. When an elderly individual was not available for an interview, or refused, another individual was randomly chosen from the list. In one instance, only one senior at a specific hotel was available. In addition, the list developed was limited by the knowledge of the management, who were sometimes uncertain of residents' ages.

The net result is that this sample is not a valid representation of *all* older SRO residents, since this approach was biased against finding certain residents, especially those who may be employed or very active. It is also less likely to pick up chronically homeless persons who use hotels only occasionally, although among both the ES and SRO samples there are seniors who have experienced homelessness at various times.

Interviewers

A total of 5 interviewers were employed (all female, four white and one black), three of whom were with the project throughout the entire interviewing phase. Their academic backgrounds included social work, sociology, and anthropology. Two of the five had doctoral degrees, two had masters degrees, and all had previous interviewing experience. Interviewers were trained in the field by the principal investigator. Interviewers worked in teams of two because it was possible to collect more complete data on the elderly individuals' current situation with one interviewer free to observe and take notes on the living conditions and the respondent's reactions to questions. Secondly, it was often necessary to search for respondents, whose last contact with ES was sometimes three or even four years before, with rare assurances that they would still be at their last known address. Due to the often dangerous nature of the neighborhoods in which respondents had lived and our lack of knowledge of the buildings being approached, teams were more appropriate for the safety of the interviewers.

SOURCES OF DATA

Agency Records

In addition to the coded information from ES records as described previously, additional descriptive client data were gathered from the client files of the DHS Youth and Family Services follow up senior unit, DAD case Management Units, and Travelers and Immigrants Aid Health Care for the Homeless (HCH) on each case where it was available. Agency records were recorded verbatim and all referrals were noted. The kind of information collected from ES records is described in Chapter 2. Additional information was gathered from conversations with agency personnel while trying to locate each individual in the interview sample.

SRO Interviews and Observations

A total of 33 hotel assessments were completed (as described in Chapters 7 and 8 in this volume), allowing a broad view of the positive and negative features of hotel living for older residents. (A copy of the assessment instrument is available upon request.) Additional information (a short questionnaire asking residents their age and why they were living in their hotel) was gathered from about 40 older residents of these same hotels.

An ethnographic approach was used with interviews of hotel managers, owners, and desk clerks. At least an hour was spent with each individual (sometimes more than once) discussing the characteristics of the hotel and it's suitability for older residents, listing the hotel's elderly residents, and describing the management's experience with them. Many other informal discussions were held in hotel lobbies, residents' rooms, and hallways with groups of residents, desk clerks, maids, bellmen and janitors.

Interviews and Observations of the Elderly

An indepth "extended client assessment" interview instrument was developed and pilot tested in June and July. This instrument combined the Duke University Older Americans Resources and Services (OARS) instrument, some questions on client background from Sosin's (1988) study of homelessness in Chicago, and the recent Ethnic Elderly Needs Assessment conducted for Chicago Department on Aging and Disability. This instrument was designed to measure the individual's health and mental health status, functional ability (ADL), social and familial support, and housing history, condition and prospects. (The interview schedule is available upon request.) Data on housing also provided a longitudinal in-depth retrospective view of the clients' residential history and gave a feel for what would happen to older adults if forced to move. The interview instrument was designed to be administered in 30-40 minutes and to stimulate narrative responses. Interviews actually lasted between 30 minutes and 1.5 hours. The same instrument was used for interviews with both SRO residents and ES clients. About two-thirds of the interviews were tape recorded and the rest were not because of either refusals or technical problems. All those interviewed, as well as other informants who provided us with extensive information, were paid $5 for their time.

Of the 115 ES cases (123 clients) chosen for interview, 94 were eventually located and a case history was completed on 91. In-person interviews were conducted with 56 clients, including formal assessments with 37. (Formal assessments could not be completed on 13 clients who were too cognitively impaired, ill, weak or unwilling.) Ancillary informants provided formal assessments on another 6 cases for a total of 43 formal assessments. In addition, ancillary informants provided useful data on 86 cases. So, in addition to the formally conducted interviews covering health, mental health, economic and social resources, a wealth of information was gathered on housing histories and lifestyles through less formal dialogue with elderly clients, family, friends, neighbors and agency sources. Fair to very complete case histories were compiled based on the combined sources of information for 91 of the 115 cases in the interview sample, resulting in an overall 79% response rate.

Interviews were also conducted with the 30 SRO residents as mentioned previously. Hotel managers, owners, desk clerks, maids, bellmen and janitors were also interviewed concerning specific elderly residents and the management's experience with them. The comparative analysis utilized only the 27 residents who were aged 60 or older.

In all interview settings, observations made by the interviewers themselves were recorded as a separate source of information. In many cases sketches or photographs of the elderly individual's private residential space were also included with the case data.

Locating the ES Clients and Variation in the Quality and Quantity of Data

Unlike street surveys or other on site random samples of the homeless, the portion of this study concerning the 115 ES clients began with a list of names of persons who had received services from ES from 1 month to 4 years in the past. The retrospective nature of these events presented significant problems for gathering data, but also provided some uniquely valuable information. Given the amount of time that had lapsed since service, the often transient housing pattern of many individuals and the lack of formal agency information regarding most of the "in need of shelter" clients, locating past clients of ES presented a challenge. Although the time varied greatly, an average of 11 hours was spent per case contacting agencies (including shelters), hospitals, the police, clients, relatives or neighbors by phone and in person. A substantial amount of this time was spent talking with relatives or persons in the neighborhood of the client's "last known address" and visiting numerous shelters and drop-in centers in efforts to locate individuals. As a result, the quality and quantity of data available on the 115 clients chosen varies, as noted previously and below.

Persistent searching for these individuals was productive in most cases and the information on these individuals is now as complete as any collected on homeless populations. In many cases it has much more depth and detail. Because of the time elapsed since ES contacts, the study provides a longitudinal view of housing patterns and experiences. The clients' own explanations and interpretations, when fit into a larger pattern of events, yield particularly richly textured explanations.

Despite the variation in the quality and quantity of data, overall it allows for richer and thicker description than anticipated. Because of the extended time spent in locating individuals we were able to contact more informants than previously anticipated and therefore collect multiple accounts of the individuals situation in many cases. However, this was not possible in every case and this variation in number and sources, as well as in the extent of and reliability of information, is a limit on the generalizability of our findings.

For example, in a few cases we were unable to contact anyone and so had to rely entirely upon already existing agency records. In other cases we were able only to contact a friend or neighbor. Yet, in a considerable number of cases we were able to collect information from the elderly client, several other informants and sometimes several agencies. In some instances, informants were particularly knowledgeable while in others very little was known about the client. This approach proved particularly valuable in accounting for clients who were deceased, institutionalized, incapacitated or otherwise uninterviewable.

Secondly, data collected from the respondents themselves, even when interviewed, was sometimes limited. In some cases the subject's state of mind (e.g., due to alcohol consumption, mental illness or dementia) precluded "accurate" accounts of the situation. In the cases where we only have the account of the elderly individual (as is the case with many SRO residents) there was no way to compare multiple accounts for discrepancies and informative incongruities. Additionally, the relationship of the interviewers to the informants sometimes affected the amount and kind of information collected. Fear, distrust, habitual "conning" or anger (at being disturbed or at being "studied") were all factors. Some informants were evasive; information given sometimes drastically contradicted other informants' accounts. Such accounts of an individual's situation (even by elderly respondents) are neither "right" or "wrong." Rather, the incongruities between accounts offer much information about the values and coping mechanisms of the respondents. Even without multiple accounts in all cases, what we have yields valuable insights.

As a result of incongruities in the data, it is necessary to make some assessment of the reliability of the information collected. The interviewer rated the general reliability of the information gathered for each individual respondent. When it was not clear which version of a fact was accurate, or when information was not given, but the interviewer had a strong hunch about it, this information was rated as questionable or unconfirmed. Unconfirmed or questionable data are not included in any analyses unless they are so labeled. Thus, if it is not clear whether the individual lived alone or with someone else, this variable was coded as unknown. If it was extremely likely that an individual had at some time been homeless, but we had no direct confirmation of this, it was coded as "suspected," but unconfirmed." Any analysis comparing those who have been homeless with those who have not been homeless was done omitting the individuals for whom the data were unconfirmed.

DATA MANAGEMENT AND ANALYSIS

As has been mentioned above, data was collected from a variety of sources. All information on interview sample respondents was kept in individual file folders and both files and tapes were given code numbers for purposes of confidentiality. Information from different sources (including agency records, phone calls and face to face conversations and interviews) was labelled as to source, date and context. The researchers' own observations were also recorded and labelled as a separate source of information.

The total sample of 475 ES cases were coded on the basis of coding in the 1987 pilot study for demographic data, the number of people in the client's household, the referral source, ES contact dates, the nature of the crises (presenting problems and other problems), living arrangements, services received and referrals made. Further coding was done on data collected from the interviews for both ES clients and SRO residents.

Several methods were utilized in coding, interpreting and analyzing the data obtained on the ES interview sample. During the course of data collection, a student working with DAD constructed detailed timelines of events for each ES client who had also been served by DAD either before or after ES contact. This indicated how and when ES, YFS and DAD referred and responded to each case. Detailed review of interviews and ancillary information on respondents was used to construct housing history timelines. These housing histories summarized in chronological order information on the timing of relocations, the reasons, household composition at each move, and any significant losses (e.g., social or economic) that coincided with them. They highlight discrepant accounts from multiple informants and denials by the interviewees. In dealing with contradictory housing history accounts with a given client, the most plausible housing history was recorded based on agreement among informants through triangulation of data sources.

REFERENCES

Douglass, R. (1988). *Aged, alone and adrift*. Detroit Area Agency on Aging.

Hoch, C. (1985). *SRO's: An endangered species*. Chicago: Community Emergency Shelter Organization and Jewish Council on Urban Affairs.

Keigher, S. (1987). *The city's responsibility for the homeless elderly*. Chicago Department of Aging and Disability.

Kutza, E. (1987). *Undomiciled elderly persons in Chicago*. Park Ridge: Retirement Research Foundation.

Rossi, P., Fisher, G. & Willis. (1986). *The condition of the homeless in Chicago*. Chicago: National Opinion Research Center.

Sosin, M., Colson, P., Grossman, S. (1988). *Homelessness in Chicago*. Chicago: The Chicago Community Trust.